Includ... ...entia
in De... ...

# Including the Person with Dementia in Designing and Delivering Care

'I Need to be Me!'

*Elizabeth Barnett*
*Foreword by Mary Marshall*

Jessica Kingsley Publishers
London and Philadelphia

Excerpt from *1,000 Airplanes on the Roof,* a science fiction music drama by Phillip Glass, text by David Henry Hwang, 1989 reproduced by kind permission of Dunvagen Music Publishers, Inc. Copyright © Dunvagen Music Publishers, Inc. Excerpt from *The Vision of Glory* by J. S. Collis, 1972, reprinted by kind permission of A. P. Watt Ltd on behalf of Michael Holroyd.

First published in the United Kingdom in 2000 by
Jessica Kingsley Publishers Ltd
116 Pentonville Road, London
N1 9JB, England
and
325 Chestnut Street
Philadelphia
PA 19106, USA.

*www.jkp.com*

**Library of Congress Cataloging in Publication Data**
A CIP catalog record for this book is available from the Library of Congress

**British Library Cataloguing in Publication Data**
A CIP catalogue record for this book is available from the British Library

ISBN 1 85302 740 5

Printed and Bound in Great Britain by
Athenaeum Press, Gateshead, Tyne and Wear

# Contents

# Acknowledgements

During the five years of this study I was most generously helped and supported by a great variety of people. My first and greatest thanks are due to the eighty-seven respondents – clients, carers, staff and managers – without whose cooperation I would have had no data to work with. Since they all received my written promise of total confidentiality I am unable to name them, but if at any time any of them should read this book I would like them to know with how much gratitude I remember each and every interview. In particular my client respondents gave me, often at the expense of considerable effort, extraordinary insight into the fundamentals of the human condition, from which I have benefited not only as a researcher but as a person.

Of those others whom I am at liberty to name, my supervisor, Linda Challis, was the companion of my eventful journey from 'having a good idea' to completing a doctoral thesis. I wish to thank her for her unwavering faith in me, especially at those times when I was unable to share it. Mary Marshall and Rik Cheston accomplished the difficult task of combining the roles of examiner, guide and friend. To Andrew Wall and Dr Mark Charny I owe my beginnings as a researcher; they provided me with the opportunities, encouragement, training and resources which came to fruition in this study. Phil Griffiths and Robin Smith were the two successive managers who guided my career development, believed in my ideas and taught me by example the creative art of management. Chris Born financed the transcription of the client interviews. Alison Middleton and Hazel May were the first to believe in the potential of my idea for using Dementia Care Mapping (DCM) as a consciousness-raising tool; and Roger Pedley supported publication.

Laura Sutton patiently taught me her innovative method, without which I could never have accessed the client perspective which came to form the basis of my study. To the late Prof. Tom Kitwood I owe not only my introduction to DCM, and personal help with data-gathering, but also my education as a DCM trainer. His encouragement and support guided me along new paths which I would otherwise never have envisaged, and on which Dawn Brooker and Jane Fossey gave me such good companionship.

To the staff of Woodbrooke College in Birmingham, where much of the data analysis was completed, and particularly to Janey O'Shea and my fellow members of 'the D-Team' go special thanks for all their faithful upholding.

To Rauf Bayraktar, Hal Laren and Betty Duke I owe the unfailing support of my own personhood and well-being; their love and patience through all the vicissitudes of five years' research make me proud to be a member of their family. And finally, to my husband and personal 'publisher of truth', Dr Perry Williams, who has lovingly accompanied me through the final critical labours of writing, I wish to dedicate this book.

*For Perry*
*without whom this book would not have been written,*
*and in memory of Tom Kitwood*

## Author's note

Managers of dementia care services, those who plan and purchase them, and those who work within them are constantly being challenged to provide more and better care within very limited resources. In evaluating these services we need to ask what we mean by 'cost', and what constitutes 'effectiveness'. Under 'cost' should we not include the emotional and psychological costs borne by all those involved? And should not 'effectiveness' by measured in terms of how closely a service approximates to the requirements of its users? Arising from a particular evaluation, this book demonstrates how we can gain access to the perspective and the lived experience of care of elderly clients with dementia, and the effect on care delivery when we do. It advocates a companionship model of care, in which the point of view of the clients is crucial, and which allows care to flow in both directions between clients and carers.

This is a book for anyone who decides on the how, what, where and when of dementia care, or is involved in the delivering of it.

# Foreword

Elizabeth Barnett is a fine advocate for people with dementia. She brings to dementia care a strong sense of justice as well as humanity and compassion. I always find that conversations with her leave pieces of grit in my mind I worry over constantly and which I find reshape my thinking in due course. I once asked her why she did not have some objective and quantifiable measures in her evaluation, such as taking the weight of the patients systematically. I think measuring weight is a useful way of knowing that basic needs are being met, at least as far as food is concerned. Without pausing for breath Elizabeth replied that she had not thought that staff would like to be weighed and she would need to use the same research approach for all participants. Another time she asked me why it might be that people could walk past someone with dementia who was expressing real emotional pain and distress without doing anything, yet the same person would be quite unable to walk past someone expressing physical pain and distress.

This passionate sense of justice imbues this lucid and thought-provoking book. The book is arguing for including people with dementia in the same model of user-based services that we want for everyone receiving help in their lives. We all want services to be based on the expressed views of users and, on the whole, people with dementia have been unheard. Elizabeth tells a story in this book, about a specialist unit called Green House. She tells us about the troubled origins and development of the unit, and about her evaluation of the care provided. The narrative enables her both to raise the issues about dementia care, and how to obtain feedback from people with dementia, and to provide real experience of how this works in practice. Her evaluation of the two dementia services provided in Green House, using interviews with all parties, including people with dementia, provides rich experience and very real voices.

This book is timely. Planners and providers are waking up to the fact that people with dementia have views and preferences if we are willing to make the effort to listen to them. This book will be a great help to them. But it will do more because it also raises a whole set of issues about dementia and dementia care which will make an invaluable contribution to our thinking.

*Professor Mary Marshall,*
*Dementia Services Development Centre*
*University of Stirling*

# Introduction

This book grew out of a particular evaluation of a new, purpose-built facility for elderly health service clients with dementia. Uniquely at the time this evaluation set out to prioritise the perspective of these clients. What came out of the evaluation has radical implications for service design and for effective practice, as well as for audit. For when we make the commitment to try to listen to what people with dementia can tell us about what is important to them, we are setting out down a road which may take us to a very different understanding, not only of the sort of services we should be designing, but also to a different model of care. Beyond that, even, we may begin to learn something about ourselves, our capabilities, and what it is to be human.

The subtitle of this book – *I Need to be Me!* – comes from words said to me by a physically disabled and very memory-impaired elderly woman who was a long-term client in the in-patient unit of the service I was evaluating, Green House. They were words said with great feeling, in the middle of a large and dreary dayroom distressingly filled with the cries and shuffling footsteps of 'wandering' lost souls. It cost her a supreme effort to find these words, and then to say them – but she was determined to convey to me her predicament, and she succeeded. I feel that she spoke for many, many others. For to my mind this phrase encapsulates perfectly the overall theme of the book: that is, the profound need to preserve the positive sense of self for which the clients I interviewed were asking. This has, therefore, to be a crucial element in caring for them – in which case we need to listen to them so as to know the person they are now. Just knowing who they were yesterday is not enough. Everyone changes and evolves throughout their life, and particularly so as a result of traumatic events. We need to learn how to follow the person through the course of their dementia: to *be* with them. Companionship has to be the key to caring.

If you have picked up this book from the shelf I think you are probably either someone who *decides* on the how, what, where and when of care, or someone who is involved in *delivering* it. If you are in the first group you may be a relative, a GP, a manager in either health or social services, a community social worker, or a community mental health worker; you may be involved in 'purchasing' care, or you may be a policy-maker. If you are in the second group you may, again, be a relative, a member of a day-care centre or day-hospital staff, a residential social worker, nurse, occupational therapist, psychologist, doctor, or one of a variety of care staff in residential or in-patient settings. You may, indeed, belong to both groups. Dementia comes close to so many people that you may be involved in dementia care in more than one capacity. Whichever perspective you come from, this book does not set out to provide easy answers. It does, however, set out to explore three questions: *Why* should we access the perspective of elderly people with dementia? *How* can we do so? *What are the implications* if we do?

At a practical level I hope that this book will help to show decision-making processes about care and services for people with dementia (the 'what' of care) as inseparable from the manner of care delivery (the 'how' of care). Both need to be rooted in a real understanding of the perspective, needs and concerns of the people for whom dementia care services are ostensibly intended: elderly clients with dementia. Yet these are the people whose point of view has for too long been missing from anyone's calculations. It is not that those who make the decisions and deliver care do not recognise the existence of their service users; but they do not recognise that they have a perspective on the care situation – that they are *aware*.

The broader debate to which this book seeks to contribute is the discussion around how we realise our accountability to those who are not themselves able to hold providers and decision-makers to account. Elderly people with dementia are not the only group who are disabled in this way. But demographic trends mean that they are becoming the largest. Therefore the ways in which society chooses to support them are going to be increasingly on the social policy agenda. Moreover, the public service sector is being driven increasingly towards a customer focus (typified by the Patient's Charter) and gathering momentum in other areas with such initiatives as 'league tables' and 'naming and shaming'. This same emphasis is moving, in the health service, through pre-occupation with 'audit' and 'advocacy' into concern with finding ways of evaluating as accurately as possible services (and the care delivered in them) to those who have not up till now been able to get their perspective taken on board. In other words, this book is part of the movement towards greater social inclusion.

I should acknowledge my own limited credentials in this area. I came to this research subject with no clinical background – in other words, I began with a thoroughly 'lay' (albeit management) perspective. My background was in health service administration, and initially I got into research through my management training. Having been commissioned to research key issues in the design of facilities for elderly people with dementia, I subsequently seized the opportunity of evaluating a brand-new, purpose-built unit, constructed as part of the re-provisioning of services from a closing old psychiatric hospital. Evaluation is a complex task, and I felt a strong ethical and intellectual need to access the views of as many as possible of the people involved with the new unit – including the clients themselves. This was several years ago, when meaningful communication with people with dementia was not usually considered possible. As we begin the twenty-first century, however, it would be nice to believe that things have changed, that attitudes are more progressive. You, the reader, can judge how far this is in fact the case from your own experience.

Why should we try to hear that elderly people with dementia can tell us about their experience? This I see as the fundamental question of the book, and so we explore it right at the beginning in Chapter One. We also explore some of the reasons why we may *not* want to try to listen to what elderly people with dementia have to tell us about the services we offer them. A brief look at the history of service provision (and non-provision!) for elderly people with dementia shows that it has been neither for, nor informed by, those people themselves. The fear of 'losing one's mind' leads us effectively to deny the continued sentient existence of those who do, with consequent deleterious effects on their well-being and sense of self. We look at the implications of the vicious circle of denial at both the individual and the societal level.

Assuming that we wish to inform our care delivery and service provision by using the perspective of service users, Chapter Two examines how we can actually do that. How can we learn to understand people with dementia? Here I look at two ways. The first is to develop an ear for metaphor, and interpret the emotional and psychological significance of memory-stories recounted by elderly people with dementia. The important thing here is that you don't have to be a practising psychotherapist to do this; you just have to be prepared to listen supportively, and open your own mind to the 'poetry', if you will, of what is being said. The second way is to look at behaviour as Tom Kitwood suggested: not as a problem to be managed but rather as meaningful communication to be read. I discuss the particular method of Dementia Care Mapping as a structured way in which to do this.

In Chapter Three I focus on the story of Green House itself. Why and how it came into being are important in understanding the service which resulted. The level of commitment to providing the best possible service for elderly people with dementia 'in the community' was remarkable, and all the more so given the background of enormous political and structural change in the health service over that period. This is a particular snapshot of the implementation of the policy of community care. Yet a certain pattern of disregard for the wishes of 'the community' is significant in light of the 'trickle-down' practice of disregard which subsequently characterised several of the relationships within the Green House service.

In Chapter Four we look at the concerns of the client respondents, which clustered into four 'meta-themes'. The first of these was their awareness – of themselves, their forgetfulness, their situation. The second was the significance for them of other people – in both positive and negative ways. The third concerned a variety of issues around the topic of loss – in particular loss of home and loved ones, or bereavement. And the final meta-theme concerned the whole question of dependence – especially its individual, subjective meanings, knowledge of which is hugely significant for those who deliver care. In particular we hear how some clients suggested that real care was about interdependence. What is more, we hear how these issues were expressed by the clients themselves – in their own words. A number of significant memory-stories show how we can extrapolate meaning through interpreting the metaphorical content in such stories. All in all, I hope that reading this chapter opens a door for the reader into ways of listening.

Given these clients' perspectives, Chapter Five moves on to look at their observed experience of care, and how this did – or did not – correlate with the pre-occupations they had expressed in their interviews. This is where we explore the results of the Dementia Care Mapping (DCM) observations, and the insights they furnished into clients' actual lived experience of care. One of the most interesting findings was the correlation between ability levels (especially verbal ability) and measured levels of well-being and ill-being. Quite simply it showed that the more able a person is, the greater their level of well-being. Not only is well-being self-supported, but it is also more rewarding for staff to work with relatively more able clients, leading to a virtuous circle. However, the opposite is also true, and there is a vicious circle of the less able whose levels of ill-being are unaddressed by those around them, leading to further deterioration.

How did those around them see things? Clearly we need to understand the views and experiences of all those involved in the service. In Chapter Six, therefore, we look at how the other groups involved (staff, carers, managers) saw things at Green House, and what lay behind their perspectives. In particular we examine the reason why no one but the client can be 'the client's voice'. For managers tend to believe that staff know about clients' needs and are their advocates; and staff believe that family carers know all about their client-relative

– their wants and needs. In fact, when we listen to individuals in all these groups we realise that everyone experiences 'dependency' in one shape or another, and that the perspective of each group is deeply affected by it. No one can 'speak for' anyone else in a situation where each group has its own vital interest.

In Chapter Seven we look at what can begin to happen when those directly involved in caring for elderly people with dementia are given the opportunity to understand their clients' experience of care. For as a direct result of using DCM in the original evaluation, the health service trust involved set up a project (which I project-managed and which included Green House) to investigate precisely this: what happens to service quality when staff and managers are given the opportunity and the skills to observe clients' actual experience of care? Accordingly a majority of hands-on staff of all disciplines and none, together with many managers and two family carers, were trained in DCM and given the opportunity to use it. Together we discovered that this led to a measurable – and very dramatic – decrease in the levels of client ill-being. In other words, through learning to read the meanings of individuals' behaviour we were able to reduce their suffering very considerably.

Finally in Chapter Eight we return to the question of why we should be seeking to access and include the views and experience of elderly clients with dementia when we design, provide and evaluate services for them. Evaluation of the quality of anything means looking at cost-effectiveness, and dementia care services are no different. But what do we mean by 'cost' and what constitutes 'effectiveness'? In the former should we not include the emotional and psychological costs borne by all those involved in the present way of organising things? And should not effectiveness be measured in terms of how closely a service approximates to the requirements of its users? Managers of services and those who plan and purchase them are constantly being challenged to provide more and better care within very limited resources, but they are also working in the dark – without realistic criteria for either prioritising or evaluation. Yet we *can* find out 'what works' for our elderly service users with dementia. Indeed, we can aim beyond the meagre aim of 'quality assurance'. into completely new pastures, where we can devise and operationalise a new, mutually rewarding and affirming companionship model of care: one in which the perspective of the clients is crucial, and which allows the care to flow both ways.

It is, therefore, the long-term aim of this book to contribute to better service provision in the future for elderly people with dementia and their carers, and a more rewarding, less frustrating working experience for hands-on care staff and the managers who support them. The use of the Green House case study is to illuminate some of the practicalities of bringing about such change, and – I hope – to stimulate further ideas in the mind of you, the reader. However, in using a case study the protection of the identities and sensibilities of past and present persons involved in it has always been a primary consideration. Future benefits do not outweigh present obligations. Consequently I have disguised both persons and places by changing the names of both, even though this has meant in many instances to deny credit where it is most abundantly due. Of all those involved in the Green House story whom I interviewed – and there were nearly a hundred of them – not one proceeded from anything other than a strong desire to do their best for the elderly clients with dementia whose service was their responsibility. This same desire informed both their participation in the research and the organisation's subsequent permission to use the story in this book. The story of Green House is a story without villains – but with many different points of view. It is a story of change. This means that what counts as enlightened, forward-thinking and innovative at any given moment in time, does not necessarily seem so to future eyes. Yesterday's innovative solution is today's taken-for-granted practice – and tomorrow's outmoded idea. Nevertheless, we should not shirk the task of our own point of history. Tomorrow may shake its head over our shortcomings; but let us at least show the future that we cared – and that we tried. This is *our* moment. Let's make it count.

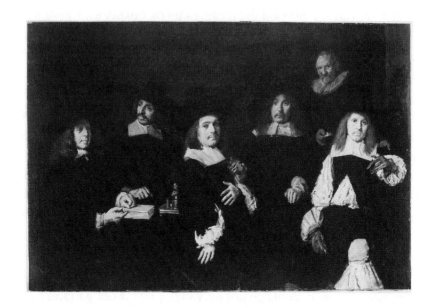

*Figure 1 'The Regents of the Old Men's Almshouse' by Frans Hals (1580–1666).*
*(Reproduced by kind permission of the Frans Halsmuseum of Haarlem, Netherlands.)*

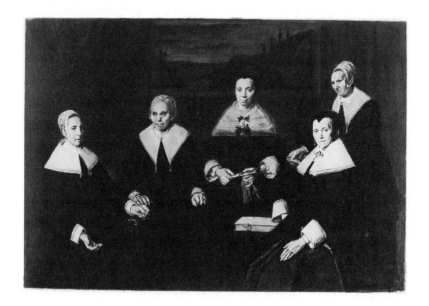

*Figure 2 'The Regentesses of the Old Men's Almshouse' by Frans Hals (1580–1666).*
*(Reproduced by kind permission of the Frans Halsmuseum of Haarlem, Netherlands.)*

# CHAPTER I

# Why listen?

*Why should we listen to the views and experience of elderly people with dementia when they are clients of our services? Have we ever done so? What are the implications of not listening?*

When age and infirmity, rather than affection and shared interest, shape relationships between people, what happens to those people? Nearly three and a half centuries ago, in 'The Regents and Regentesses of the Old Men's Almshouse', the painter Frans Hals set down on canvas a rare insight into this kind of relationship from the perspective of the frail and powerless elderly recipient (Figs. 1 and 2). Although this is a book specifically about elderly people with dementia, and we have no record of such a diagnosis being attributed to Hals himself, nevertheless his pictorial record of experience of the 'care' relationship of his day still has something particularly pertinent to say about care provision for frail elderly people – mental frailty being considered the most extreme infirmity in our society.

When he painted these portraits Hals was well into his eighties, utterly destitute, and dependent on the charity of his 'local authority'. Whether as a gesture of gratitude or because they required it, he painted the portraits of the Regents and Regentesses who administered alms to him. These pictures are disturbingly honest portrayals of the faces of 'care' in the late seventeenth century. For they do not exactly radiate compassion and sensitivity. There is not, for example, a single smile among them. They turn towards the painter a cool, disinterested regard, devoid of human warmth. And the hands are strikingly emblematic of how Hals experienced the dependent relationship. Portraying hands is one of the most difficult challenges for a representational artist, so Hals was showing the painterly skills he still retained. But the hands he painted were not generous or giving. One woman has her hand outstretched (just) towards the painter, but the gesture is stiff and grudging. As for the man who is pointing directly towards the painter, his hand is depicted like a claw. In each picture the sitters are grouped around a prominent book. Would this have been a bible, or an accounts ledger? That is, was it the symbol of the cultural imperative for their assistance, or the calculated record of their generosity? Alms-giving is shown as a cold ethic. This is indeed a compelling image of 'charity' in its fully pejorative sense: 'charity' which gives practical assistance (in Hals' case, food and fuel) but takes away – 'claws back' – self-respect.

Hals has shown us with depressing clarity the stiff, unbending emotional deformity which the 'care' relationship he experienced created in the givers. By his very skill in portraying of it he has also shown us something else: that, destitute, frail, elderly and dependent though he was, he yet retained the capabilities which had made him a great artist: clarity and insightfulness of observation, and honesty and skilfulness of expression. In other words, he still had a point of view, and the ability to express it. We can wonder whether his sitters were receptive to the perspective he offered them. What did they do with this unusual opportunity of 'feedback' which his portraits afforded them?

What would we do if an elderly person with dementia were to offer us an analogous opportunity? Would we, indeed can we, as Faith Gibson recently asked, 'risk person-centred communication' with the person with dementia? (Gibson 1999). What might happen if we did? This book is about a piece of research that tried to do exactly this, by seeking to evaluate a brand-new, purpose-built unit for elderly health-service clients with dementia, within their own terms and their own experience. The findings suggest that in 'hearing the voice of people with dementia' (Goldsmith 1996) we hear voices proceeding not from an altogether different set of values than those of us, as it were, as yet without dementia, but where the values are ranked in a different order of priority. We might put it another way and say that those of us, as it were, without dementia have a tendency to concentrate on the expression of our values (such as privacy, choice, dignity), whereas a person with dementia tends to focus on the source, the fundamentals of living and relating.

It is interesting that communicating with elderly people with dementia has for so long been considered at best problematic, and most often impossible. For the communication barrier is not usually erected by the person with dementia.

> You're very welcome to ask me at any time for what I know might be very helpful. If there's anything you want to learn about from me, you're welcome.

Thus an elderly person attending a day-hospital for people with dementia greeted my request for an interview to find out about his experience there. In fact, of the two-thirds of all the people attending the day-hospital or its attached in-patient facility whom I approached, not one refused the opportunity to be interviewed about their views of the service. Many of them showed their understanding of the interview situation by referring to it directly during the course of the interview. They knew their views were being canvassed, and they were 'very glad to be of help.' One man explained: 'I know quite a lot really – so I would appreciate the fullest confidence.' (Did he 'really' mean 'confidentiality', or did he really mean 'confidence' – that is, that I should trust his ability?) And another, newly recovering from a major stroke, was concerned to emphasise that 'Most people, you know, I expect you find, are so bright. People are brighter than we think ... Give them half a chance, they can be resourceful, they can be helpful.'

Why should we be trying to hear what elderly people with dementia can tell us about their experiences of care in the services run ostensibly for them? This is the fundamental question with which this book is concerned. The person who believed in the capabilities of each individual ('people are brighter than we think'), and that therefore, if given the opportunity, 'they can be helpful', was also the person who continued his line of thought by making the case for a more egalitarian practice of 'care': 'You don't have to bend down on people, not that at all, no. It's give and take. Yes, I love that – give and take.' Why should we be interested in such a idea?

First, we might consider the implications of completing, or not completing, the feedback loop of service provision and care delivery for people with dementia. We seek feedback from users of other services (be they supermarkets or hospitals) so why not from people with dementia? Are they non-persons? For there are other people in our society who are similarly often not counted as full members, with a right to be consulted, informed and involved in decisions affecting their lives – for instance, those who are seen as not yet ready (because of their youth) or equipped (because of disability) for social member- ship, and those whose misdemeanours have led to their forfeiting such membership (prisoners). So this phenomenon of being locked out of the consultation process is not unique to people with dementia. However, noting with whom we implicitly classify them is revealing of some of our attitudes towards people with dementia. It betrays not only our condescension and our infantilisation of them (the 'second childhood' concept), but also our disapproval of their behaviour and our horror of, and distancing ourselves from, their cognitive incom- petencies.

This exclusion of people with dementia from the feedback loop in evaluating care provision has the consequence that service providers and policy-makers rely on the views of those accepted as proxy voices for service users. Thus relatives and caregivers are considered adequate advocates for people with dementia, without recognising that each of these groups will necessarily have an agenda of their own. This situation is only beginning to change:

The 1990 NHS and Community Care Act requires service providers to consult with their consumers about the services they would wish to receive. In the field of dementia care, the carer has been perceived as being the consumer. This view is now being questioned. In order to improve services for people with dementia and to make them more responsive to individual need it is necessary first to accept that they have a voice, second to facilitate the use of that voice, and third to hear it. (Goldsmith 1996, p.161)

The second reason for seeking the perspective of clients with dementia is the classic one of quality assurance: we need to incorporate user perspectives in order to ensure that resources are being utilised with maximum effectiveness. Indeed, we require access to this perspective in order to determine in the first instance what constitutes effectiveness. In other words, without the user perspective how can we know what it is that we should be measuring? This highlights the slippery slope down which the acceptance of proxy voices pushes us. For if we have set our service and care objectives informed by other agendas than those of the people for whom the service is ostensibly and ultimately intended, then we will have no way of knowing whether the effort, money, and initiative expended is in fact 'hitting the spot'. There is a destructive circular logic to this process. The more we listen to other voices, the less we will be able to hear the voice of the elderly client with dementia. Although involving family carers in decisions about their incapacitated loved one is clearly a good thing, it can lead to an insidious slide into a self-perpetuating circle of mutual reassurance that everything possible is being done for the client. But does the client think so?

This brings us to the third reason for seeking feedback. We are not wrong to seek reassurance and satisfaction that we are meeting our objectives and obligations. But believing that we cannot get this from people with dementia themselves has enervating and disempowering consequences for everyone concerned. We need to establish communication with those for whom we are caring, for both personal and professional reasons. For we need to understand our task better, so that we may learn, and enrich our experience and understanding. In pushing back the frontiers of our understanding we can cease to be at the mercy of that which we cannot comprehend. Rather, we can find ways of taking charge, of addressing the enormous challenge of dementia.

This is where the so-called 'medical model' of dementia is unhelpful. If we view dementia only as a 'disease', then we are tempted to abdicate our fundamental responsibility as human beings for the welfare of our fellows, and leave it to scientists in laboratories to discover the pill, potion, gene or magic bullet that will 'treat' or even 'cure' dementia. But if we see dementia as a condition of which organic degenerative brain disorder is only one part, but which is also fuelled by the fear, anxiety, shame, and incomprehension of both the person concerned, those with whom they are in contact, and the wider society in which we all have our being – then we can begin to see that we have a role to play ourselves. The consequence of such a view of dementia is empowering for all concerned; we all have the possibility to feel better about ourselves. After all, do we want to feel that all we can do is be custodians of those who are no longer quite human? In expanding our model of dementia we return humanity and self-respect both to those 'with' dementia and those 'without' it. For this view of dementia recognizes a dislocation of relationship, triggered by brain dysfunction in one person and fuelled by fear, in them and everyone else.

In discovering the abilities of the person with dementia for whom we care, we also discover abilities (perhaps hitherto unsuspected) within ourselves. For instance, here is a 'Tale of Two Happier Men'. A skilled and experienced nurse (we will call him Paul) dreaded the daily round of intimate care with a certain elderly man with dementia, who remained hunched, silent, and seemingly insensible in his chair all day. We will call him Joe. Yet Joe roused in bathroom and bedroom to resist violently any assistance with intimate tasks of self-care, often hitting and biting staff members. After being given the opportunity to spend a shift observing the minutiae of Joe's experience in the day-room of the ward, Paul read the utter dejection of his body language, and realised the affront he must feel that the only personal attention he ever received was in the toilet or in dressing. So he decided to talk. He talked to Joe quietly and regularly, trying to convey that he understood something of how Joe might be feeling. Joe remained slumped in his wheelchair, but the hitting and biting ceased. One day Paul came running out of the ward, his face alight with amazement and joy. He had just helped Joe to bed. 'Joe talks!' he cried. Not only did Paul no longer suffer painful physical attacks, but he had discovered a new professional potential of insight and skill as a nurse. Thereafter Joe would talk (and even smile) quietly in the privacy of his bedroom or the bathroom. And Paul found increasing personal and professional satisfaction in his ability to make personal contact with the most handicapped and withdrawn people in his care.

There is a further dimension to the need for caregivers to communicate with those with dementia. It relates to the fact that long-term memories remain accessible to those with memory impairment even when short-term memory fails. Thus experiences of earlier life can remain vivid, and inform the way the present is perceived. Not all these memories are pleasant and, as higher intellectual controls atrophy, those memories that have been long repressed may surface with all the power of freshly experienced pain, shame or fear. Although not describing this phenomenon specifically in dementia, the playwright David Henry Hwang conveys it well:

> Layers upon layers of mesh. Each layer, a screen holding a memory. Some memories, easier to touch. These, put up front, on display. Behind them, others – of shame and violation and pain – these, left in obscure places, far back as possible. Yet their presence bleeds through. So that the viewer, casually perusing the collection, is disturbed, a chill runs through his body. For even as he gazes at the most ordinary of memories, he becomes aware of other images he is not supposed to see. In this way, the screens behind acquire a power greater than those in front. The room is

saturated with the presence of things hidden. (Hwang 1989, p.23)

These 'screens behind' do, indeed, acquire great power, as they can form the lens through which an elderly person with dementia perceives their environment and those within it. Their subjective world is then 'saturated with the presence of things hidden'. If we are unaware of these things, we are working in the dark. For we can be the unwitting heirs of feelings from the experiences of people with dementia resulting from the last time they were in a dependent role, that is, in childhood. Other researchers (for instance, Miesen 1992) have noted the prevalence of childhood memories of the parental relationship, recounted by elderly people with dementia in formal care settings. Some of these memories may be highly disturbing – of abuse, violence, and fear – and the need to repress them may be such that the client may never have spoken of them, even (indeed, particularly) to loved ones. Not all relevant information – especially emotional information – can be gathered by interviewing close relatives, no matter how diligent the care worker. Here again, the insufficiency of listening only to proxy voices is demonstrated. We need to understand the subjective scene upon which we enter as actors, if we are to begin to relate with understanding to those with dementia. And this implies that we should recognise the validity of that subjective scene, its 'real-ness.' How can anyone know what subjective world they are working within if they are not listening to the client directly?

Finally, and beyond these practical considerations, elderly people with dementia may tell us something about what it means to be a human being, beyond our accepted cognitive definition. They can tell us about what the essentials are when levels of 'higher' functioning are taken away, about who we are when we cannot find the words, cannot remember the place, do not recognise the person, forget what we were just saying, and lose control of our bodily functions. Do we really believe that human beings are only language-processers, place-locators, visitor-identifiers and bladder-controllers? When we are left alone with the subjective world of feelings and direct, unmediated experience, when we are caught in an eternal present – who and what are we? Thus listening to the experience of people with dementia confronts us with the big metaphysical questions with which humankind has wrestled for millennia. Perhaps we do not want to leave the shelter of confident superiority with which our neo-cortical functioning seems to provide us. We do not want to confront our own limitations, we do not want to hear that

> we are all frail people, vulnerable and wounded: it is just that some of us are more clever at concealing it than others! ... The world is not divided into the strong who care and the weak who are cared for. We must each in turn care and be cared for, not just because it is good for us, but because that is the way things are. The hardest thing for those of us who are professional carers is to admit that we are in need, peel off our sweaty socks and let someone else wash our dirty blistered feet ... It is easy to forget that so much caring, so much serving is done by people who are weary and in some way not quite whole. (Cassidy 1988, p.78)

Have we ever been prepared to listen? The research with which this book is concerned relates to an evaluation of a new, purpose-built health-service facility to provide care in the community for elderly people with dementia, which opened its doors in January 1991. We shall call it Green House. It was set in a small market town, and was part of the reprovision of mental health services from one of the old psychiatric hospitals which was being closed. But what was the historical background of care provision for elderly people with dementia, against which Green House and its evaluation need to be seen? Let us review this with particular reference to whether or not the voices of service users themselves have ever been acknowledged.

For well over a century, first the Poor Law and then the Welfare State resulted in effectively the same provision for elderly people seriously disabled with dementia: either they were cared for by relatives at home, or they were cared for in, first, the workhouse hospital or, subsequently, the geriatric wards of NHS hospitals. As many of the NHS hospitals were inherited from former workhouses it often happened (and still does) that elderly health-service patients with dementia are cared for in exactly the same buildings as their forebears under the Poor Law. For whom was Poor Law 'care' actually being provided? In enclosing the indigent poor (inevitably including those too old and frail to work) in workhouses, society demonstrated that it was effectively caring for the sensibilities of the middle class, by relieving them of the distasteful sights of poverty, starvation and disease. Those with economic and political power exercised it for their own benefit, and the mask of altruism served to bolster their belief in the rightness and propriety of their actions. How have things changed since then?

In fact, the main focus of the Welfare State in its early years was on services for mothers and children, adult health, and retirement pensions. Elderly people with dementia who had neither relatives able and willing to help them, nor independent financial resources to purchase care, were not even recognised as a separate group with specific needs, but lumped together with all 'who by reason of age, infirmity or other circumstances are in need of care and attention which is not otherwise available to them' (Section 21 of the National Assistance Act 1948). In its generality this catch-all clause is reminiscent of the undefined references to the 'indigent *poor*' of the Poor Law, where the very lack of specification itself betrays the attitude of the legislators. In other words, the defining characteristic of those referred to was their poverty and their inability to work and therefore earn. The reasons for this inability were clearly irrelevant and uninvestigated.

Although the work of Townsend (1962) and Titmuss (1961) in the sixties at last put care for the frail elderly explicitly on the social policy agenda, the economic restrictions caused by the 1974 oil crisis robbed the post-Seebohm (1968) era of its potential efficacy in this area. It was not until the late seventies and early eighties that the demographic pressure – and concomitant implications – of the 'greying' population began to be officially recognised. Also at this time the political focus was on rolling back state intervention wherever possible and ensuring cost-effectiveness of services either directly managed, or purchased, by the state. The eighties and early nineties witnessed an era where the shape of services even for the weakest and least articulate were considered to benefit from the hidden hand of market forces. Thus the recognition of resource constraints and of demographic pressures fuelled an ideological commitment to value for money. The positive side of this was the focus on quality issues and, through this, on the client-as-customer. The difficulty with regard to our client group was that the 'customer' was not seen as capable of expressing opinions or exercising choice.

This brings us back to an inherent problem of the so-called 'medical model' of dementia. For where dementia is viewed as a disease suffered by a patient, rather than a neurologically triggered but socially constructed condition which challenges not only the individual but all those around them, as well as society as a whole, issues of resource constraints can easily justify shuffling off responsibility for that which is 'incurable', and the impetus for care provision rests only upon the sense of decency of those concerned. And there is a world of difference between care that is provided because we relate to, identify with, and communicate with the recipient as someone whose problems we understand or can imagine, and care that is provided solely so that we – society in general and caregivers in particular – do not feel bad about ourselves, and can continue to respect ourselves as humane and responsible citizens.

All of this grows in large measure from the problems of communication which dementia brings with it. When we do not understand the person with dementia, it is easy to attribute this to their 'disease'. This in turn makes it seem to us that there is no possibility of communication across the divide of neurological impairment, and from this it is but a small step to denying the continued existence in real terms of the 'person' with dementia. This is the 'death-which-leaves-the-body-behind' school of thought. Consequently health service policy that has been informed by the medical model focused on the provision of day-hospitals for assessment, and limited in-patient provision for longer client assessments and 'respite' for family carers. At a time of increasing resource consciousness and focus on the client-as-customer (as, for instance, in the Patient's Charter), long-stay care for elderly clients with dementia was conveniently removed from the health service agenda, on the grounds that where no treatment or cure could be provided, all that they required was so-called 'social care.'

Through all this the personal viewpoint of the elderly man or woman with dementia has been strikingly absent. In other words, their perspective has never informed central policies, service provision, or the manner of care delivery. Theirs is the absent voice throughout all policy and service discussions and documentation. Services are set up ostensibly *for* them; we know of their existence. Yet theirs is a spectral presence, an unsettling silence at the heart of both policy and service arenas. Family carers and healthcare professionals clamour for recognition and resources. There are no demonstrations, campaigns or letters to the paper from clients themselves.

Yet the picture is not without hope. It is reassuring that over precisely this period there has arisen a growing awareness of, and interest in, dementia. In parenthesis at this point it is necessary to clarify that the dementia with which we are concerned here is that arising from primary degenerative organic brain disorder occurring – for the most part – in the population over sixty-five. In received terminology, the majority of these fall into the diagnostic categories of Alzheimer's disease or multi-infarct dementia, with a minority related to Parkinson's disease. Terminology, in fact, is a useful guide in charting the progress of our understanding of dementia. For example, we have long since moved on from using the term 'senile', with its strong flavour of contempt. The 'senile' belonged in the workhouse, or later in the 'funny farm', the asylum. Since the 1960s, terminology has reflected the increased care for, and interest in, elderly people with dementia. 'Psycho-geriatric' was initially much in favour, removing dementia from the pejorative realm of 'senility'. It is conclusively a technical, medical term, neatly classifying the person thus described as a 'patient' suffering from a condition, and therefore rightly admitting them into the domain of professional medicine. In other words, they were no longer 'mad' but 'ill'. As psycho-geriatrics grew as a specialism, a new term for dementia came into use: elderly severely mentally ill – or ESMI. Interestingly, patients, beds and whole wards shared the same acronym, whose only initial benefit was that, as an acronym, it was esoteric and therefore provided a spurious protection from stigma.

However, this was closely followed in the eighties by a more gentle and caring preference for referring to the 'confused elderly,' or the 'very frail elderly', as the increasing numbers of elderly people with dementia began to make their mark on the consciousness of service providers, who at the same time were being required to plan services 'in the community', as opposed to hidden away in the large old Victorian psychiatric hospitals. As the voices of family carers began to be raised, through organisations such as the Alzheimer's Disease Society, the terminology acquired a compassionate lilt, and 'dementia sufferer' or 'Alzheimer's sufferer' acknowledged clients' anguish. Today, we prefer simply to say 'person with dementia', which has the great advantage of putting the person first (Kitwood 1997).

Indeed, it is the emergence of the personhood of those with dementia which has been the crucial development of recent years. Since the 1960s caregivers and researchers have evolved a variety of approaches to dementia care, implicit in which has been a broader, more inclusive and more practically fruitful model of dementia (Holden and Woods 1995). These include, among others, reality orientation, reminiscence work, validation therapy and resolution therapy. Discovering the significance of various kinds of care input in achieving change for people with dementia led not only to recognition of the importance of care practices, but also to a new understanding of dementia. For the implications of the significant potential of the care input raised both questions and answers about the dementia process, including the 'pathogenic' function of poor care practice. So these new approaches represented for the first time a recognition that people with dementia are not unaware of their surroundings or unresponsive to caregivers' initiatives. More recently there has even been work on 'rementia', which confirms that people with dementia, given appropriate support, can learn and adjust, despite degenerative neurological impairment (Kitwood 1995; Sixsmith, Stilwell and Copeland 1993).

Over the past generation, therefore, there has accumulated a growing body of work, both practical and academic, which sees dementia as something infinitely more complex even than the mysteries of neuropathology. In contrast to the hopelessness engendered by the latter, a desire to understand the experience of the individual with dementia and to work with that reality has gathered momentum.

In light of this growing recognition of the personhood (Kitwood 1997) and the possibility of hearing the voice of people with dementia (Goldsmith 1996), what are the implications for all of us of *not* listening, both at the personal and the societal level? We should recall the meaning of the word: 'de-mentia'. Chambers Dictionary defines it as 'out of one's mind', 'the failure or loss of mental powers'. And we should recall also that in our culture we define ourselves as *homo sapiens*, which the same dictionary translates as 'intelligent, able to reason, man'. That is, we define ourselves as a species by our cognitive abilities.

That this way of conceiving ourselves as human beings is a cultural phenomenon rather than a universal truth has been pointed out by anthropologists and social constructionists:

> In the West, in our everyday, practical talk about ourselves, we take a great number of things for granted. And in our traditional forms of inquiry into ourselves and the nature of our everyday social lives ... we have codified these 'basic' ways of talking into a number of explicit assumptions ... Other peoples seem to have developed very different ways of accounting for themselves to each other: as Lienhardt (1961: 149) reports for the Dinka, for instance, that they seem to have 'no such interior entity [as a 'mind'] to appear, on reflection, to stand between the experiencing self at any given moment and what is or has been an

exterior influence upon the self.' Could it be that our talk of people as having inner mental states, and of them as always understanding things in terms of such states, is less universal than we think? (Shotter 1993, pp. 4–5)

Nevertheless, universal or not, that is our assumption, that is how we see ourselves, and that is the basis for our interrelating. It follows, therefore, that the loss of what we consider to be our defining characteristic (our 'core capability,' that which differentiates us from all other species) will rank among the most devastating calamities that can happen to us. The thought that such a calamity could happen to us is unbearable, and the consideration of how, if it did happen, we might feel as we experienced that-which-we-believe-actually-makes-us-human being stripped away from us, is fearful beyond measure. Therefore we have a powerful need to believe that if we lose our cognitive abilities we will not know what is happening to us. We need to believe that we will exist in a kind of living anaesthesia. It would be too awful to contemplate how one could be 'out of one's mind' and conscious of it.

However understandable this need to deny awareness in dementia, we nevertheless have to recognise how this very denial fuels and per-petuates the fear which provokes it. We can see the vicious circle of denial operating at both the individual and the societal level. At the individual level, by denying awareness of the person with dementia we are allowed to treat them as non-persons. This leads to low quality of care, which in its turn leads to the 'confused,' 'challenging,' 'demented' behaviour (for instance, the 'wandering', the constant shouting) which fuels and increases our own fear of dementia. For at some level we must be asking ourselves how we might behave if this should happen to us – and how we might be treated. Seeing the awful prospect of the poor care scenario which would await us is so terrifying that this leads to further denial. So at the individual level the vicious circle of denial has at least an apparent short-term merit in safeguarding our sanity. However, breaking the circle by accepting the awareness of people with dementia, and consequently treating them with the sensitivity we reserve for those with whom we can identify, would set up a virtuous circle. The quality of care would improve enormously, and we might then be able to contemplate the prospect of our own future experience of dementia with less fear, secure in the knowledge that we would still be loved and respected for ourselves, listened to and accepted. Much of our fear of dementia has to relate to the way in which we see people with dementia being treated.

Whereas at the individual level the vicious circle of denial relates to fear and guilt, at the societal level it revolves around resource allocation. Since labour costs always represent far and away the greatest revenue expenditure of any health or 'care' service, in times of resource consciousness labour-intensive solutions tend to be strongly resisted. This is also why those who spend the most time with the client are paid the least: in order to minimise costs. This means that the least qualified, least trained and least recognised care staff deliver the most care; for those with qualifications and training attract correspondingly higher rewards in terms of both pay and status. (Here again the concept of *homo sapiens* sets the value standard: the more *sapiens*, the more *homo*, as it were.) This lack of training and support for those who spend the most time with elderly clients with dementia in our services communicates to them unmistakably the lack of recognition of the difficult yet profoundly important nature of their work. And, despite remarkable and humane exceptions, it tends to have as its direst consequence the lack of insightful care, where insight is most needed:

> There are two common misapprehensions when discussing the voice of the people with dementia. One is that you cannot communicate with them because the nature of their illness means that they are unable to reflect or communicate. The second is that we know what they want to communicate, and without realising it, slant or coax or ask leading questions so that people with dementia who are more influenced by feelings than by facts will give the answers which they perceive we want them to give. Ascertaining their views can be a very demanding and skilful job

and those who have the responsibility for doing it need a great deal of empathy and training. As things are at the moment, the people with the most time and the greatest opportunities to do this tend to be the least trained and the least influential in making decisions about services. (Goldsmith 1996, p.164)

So this lack of insightful care, not surprisingly, leads to 'behaviour problems,' as clients react to their demotion from the world of persons to the world of objects – for that is what the denial of their subjective experience effectively means. And so the sadly familiar picture of the 'wandering,' shouting, rocking, or completely 'switched off' behaviour of clients and the insensitivity of those around them fuels our fearful perception of dementia, and leads to further denial. What is more, this denial is buttressed most conveniently by the perennial concern with resource constraints. It is so much easier to accept what appears to be the case: that people with dementia are, in some sense, not really persons any more and that therefore there is nothing very much that we can do for them. Our services, therefore (like those of the Poor Law of our forebears), are delivered to ourselves: to alleviate our own sensibilities, and to permit us not to see ourselves as uncaring or insensitive.

But let us examine the resource allocation issue again. It is founded on the concept of cost-effectiveness. It is the contention of this book that we need to reconsider both what we mean by 'effective,' and what we count as a 'cost.' The present system is far from low-cost, either in financial or in psychological terms. And the level of dissatisfaction and downright suffering of clients, carers, staff and service managers would seem to call into question its effectiveness in terms of delivering much that is positive to the well-being of anyone involved. Here it is also worth recalling the 'quick fix' nature of our contemporary western culture. We no longer have the ability to wait; pills are preferable to nursing time. So we willingly expend millions on research into future treatments and cures for neurological impairment for those in the future, yet begrudge our time (in terms of valuable person-hours) to alleviate the fear and isolation of those with dementia already amongst us. This is yet another reason why we prefer to construct dementia as a disease, rather than a dislocation of relationship.

However, if we do choose to challenge the old assumptions and move beyond our restricted conceptions of humanity, dementia, and cost-effectiveness, a new world awaits us:

> Above all else, the reconsideration of dementia invites us to a fresh understanding of what it is to be a person. The prevailing emphasis on individuality and autonomy is radically called into question, and our true interdependence comes to light. Frailty, finitude, dying and death are rendered more acceptable; grandiose hope for technical Utopias are cut to the ground. Reason is taken off the pedestal that it has occupied so unjustifiably, and for so long; we reclaim our nature as sentient and social beings. Thus from what might have seemed the most unlikely quarter, there may emerge a well-spring of energy and compassion. And here, in comparison to conventional psychiatry, we may find an immeasurably richer conception of the healing of the mind. (Kitwood 1997, p.144)

# CHAPTER 2

# How can we listen?

*How can we learn to understand people with dementia? We can find ways of listening to the words that are said, and of reading the behaviour which we see. These are not new skills, but rather an active switching on of skills we already possess.*

Goethe said that it was no use trying to wrest the truth of nature by using the screws and levers of science – we can only get out the facts that way. To get at the truth, the significances, the quality, we need another instrument. The spanner we need for that is imagination. Science tells us how things are assembled; imagination deals with the value and significance of the assembly. (Collis 1972, p.73)

## Introduction

To travel across the mountain range of denial which the limitations of our present understanding represent, into the country of the 'new culture of dementia care' (Kitwood and Benson 1995), we need to find vehicles capable of helping us across this difficult and challenging terrain. And just as transport technology evolves, so will our insight into ever better ways of interpreting and communicating with those whose cognitive deterioration presents us with such a challenge. In this chapter I will be describing two methods which I found to be particularly helpful in my own attempt to evaluate a particular dementia care facility from the perspective of its clients. I do not suggest that these are the only methods. But I do believe that it is only by beginning to use the methods which we have that new ones will evolve. And the advantage of the two methods which I shall describe is that they exploit existing human skills. That is, we need not so much to learn new skills, as not to switch off existing ones when we enter a dementia care environment.

If, therefore, we do decide to try to listen to what elderly people with dementia can tell us about the services we say we run for them, in practical terms how can we do this? This was the problem which confronted me back in 1991 when I came to evaluate a new purpose-built facility for elderly people with dementia called Green House. The story of how both Green House and my evaluation of it came about belongs to the next chapter. However, it is on this experience that I want to draw in looking at some of the methods available, the insights which can be drawn from them, and the sort of results which using them can have. The important thing to understand is that it is possible to make a well-supported imaginative leap into the world of an elderly person with dementia, and that it is not necessary to be a highly qualified clinical practitioner in order to be able to do so. When I began my evaluation of Green House I was a junior manager in the health service, with an administrative, not a clinical, background.

When I began to think about how I was going to conduct the evaluation, from the outset I wanted to include the perspective of service users. It seemed to me not only that there was an intellectual and an ethical imperative to do so – these were, after all, the people for whom the service was supposed to exist – but also that the balance of history needed to be redressed. Facilities for those with dementia had always been evaluated against criteria set up by those, as it were, without dementia. And I was aware that there could not be just *one* Green House, but many – as many, indeed, as there were people involved with it in whatever capacity, including the clients for whose benefit the service was apparently being run. The challenge, therefore, for me was how to capture as multi-dimensional a picture of the new service as possible, one in which every perspective of Green House was acknowledged.

I therefore decided to try to capture the viewpoint of the four main 'stakeholder groups' of Green House: the staff who worked there, the managers who had set it up and were responsible for running it, the family carers of those who attended it, and the service users themselves. Accessing the perspective of people in the first three groups did not appear to be problematic. I decided to interview them, using an interview schedule as a guide to the topics on which I wished to canvass their views. These would therefore be semi-structured, in-depth interviews of the type familiar in much management or social policy research. But how to access the perspective of the service users in this particular case, where failing memory and its resulting confusion and even dysphasia seemed to threaten to vitiate any such attempt? Perhaps particularly as a non-clinician I was overcome with the seeming impossibility of the task.

It was at this point that I was introduced to two people who had confronted this problem and found each their own (albeit partial) solution. The first was Laura Sutton and the second was Tom Kitwood. Laura introduced me to her own particular method of inter-viewing elderly people with dementia, and Tom to his newly evolving (at that time) observational technique which sought to 'read' the behaviour of elderly people with dementia as meaningful com-munication. Both of these methods were very new at the time I came across them; I was, in fact, one of the first (apart from their inventors) to use them. It felt as if we were travelling into terra incognita: strange, uncharted territories where previous certainties seemed insecure, and unquestioned assumptions disintegrated in a mist of new possibilities. Tom and Laura both took me on a voyage of discovery. The Green House which by that time I thought I knew, turned out to be an altogether different place, and what is more, one whose existence I had not even suspected. Like Mary in Frances Hodgson Burnett's *The Secret Garden*, I found a door into an overgrown space where what had been planted in the past now grew unchecked and unnoticed, enclosed behind high walls of ignorance, fear and neglect.

Before we explore these methods and how I used them in more depth, a word is needed about my objective of taking as egalitarian an approach as possible to the evaluation of Green House. This did not entail my employing the same methods of inquiry across all stake-holder groups. I think that when we look at services for people with whom, for whatever reason, we experience problems of communication, we need to beware a spurious egalitarianism which seeks to apply monoform data collection techniques regardless of ability or disability, thereby apparently emphasising disability, and also increasing the invisibility of the group concerned by ruling them out of the process for no better reason than their not fitting in with an arbitrary standard. If the objective of an evaluation is to access people's views and concerns, then the onus is surely upon the more 'competent' partner (that is, the partner with the greater range of communication tools) in the communication process to find those ways which will furnish possibilities for common understanding. Thus I used Laura's interviewing technique, which did not apply a schedule of topics and questions, but sought to follow deeper processes of association, memory and metaphor, which, as I discovered, we all share, to uncover the concerns of those who could not voice them directly. Similarly with regard to Tom's observational tool – Dementia Care Mapping – I did not apply analagous observa-tional methods to the staff, the managers or family carers. Since they and I were able to converse without impediment about the issues around their experience of Green House, minute-by-minute individual observations of them would have been unnecessarily, and therefore unjustifiably, intrusive. I could justify this for elderly clients with dementia only because they were the only means available to me at that time for understanding the reality of their daily experience of the service.

# Interviews

At the outset I was aware that I needed to find a way of talking to the clients of the service. My main worry was my own inexperience. For a start I had never conducted a major evaluation before. I also realised that I would probably have to acquire from scratch some very special skills, due to my lack of clinical background. In some ways, this anxiety was misplaced. I discovered that the highly individual and selective nature of cognitive impairment in what we call dementia meant that many of the day-hospital clients at Green House were able (and very willing!) to converse on a variety of topics. This was all the more true given the wide variety of their individual backgrounds. Therefore, although they were often unable to say which day it was, or even which year, they could discuss their feelings and attitudes. Most significantly also, they would enrich the conversation with examples from their past experiences – which were sometimes more vivid than recent ones. In fact, it was from this phenomenon of vivid memory-stories that the interviewing method benefited particularly.

However, the first important discovery I made was that, far from being unable to express their views directly, many of the less cognitively impaired day-hospital clients were able to contribute significant and highly personal information about their feelings, attitudes and perceptions. As the evaluation progressed, however, I found I was interviewing increasingly dysphasic and confused clients, and it was here that the significance of their memories became of particular interest. For Green House served a range of clients, from those who were mildly confused through to those who were as severely impaired as it is possible to be. When I looked back on the total of over thirty clients who at that time used both day-hospital and in-patient services at Green House, I was amazed to discover that I had been able to interview twenty-two of them – that is, approximately two-thirds.

So how did I learn how to interview elderly people with dementia? A colleague of mine had put me in touch with Laura Sutton, a clinical psychologist, who worked with elderly clients with dementia and was pioneering a research method for accessing their views and feelings. So I went to spend some time with Laura, learning about her interviewing techniques and even being allowed to sit in as an observer during some of her interviews. I learned that she worked on the principle that even where a person's levels of intellectual functioning were deteriorating through neurological impairment, their level of emotional functioning was unimpaired, although the control normally exercised over the emotions might be undermined. Interviewing someone with dementia, therefore, was about seeking to access the emotional level more directly, without relying on the usual 'rational' processes of questions and answers turn by turn. In this way people with dementia could communicate what they were feeling, what they needed, and what was important to them. But because neurological impairment is highly individually specific, each individual will find their own way to express themselves. So the interviewer's job was to facilitate this as best they could, by starting the ball rolling, as it were, with the main question in which they were interested, and then turning the agenda over to the respondent (Sutton and Fincham 1994).

Laura's method was based on certain ways of using our understanding of memory and memory-loss. The short-term memory loss suffered by those with dementia meant that they might be unable to remember or refer to events of the here-and-now, but the feelings they had about these events were still there and could be expressed, often by using long-term episodic memories as metaphors and analogies for present experiences. Hence, for example, when Laura asked an elderly dementia sufferer about his memory, he referred to his memory as a 'disaster'. And he then went on to describe many of the other disasters of his earlier life and how he had felt about them. So by analogy he was expressing his present feelings about his memory-loss and his resulting confusion (Sutton 1993).

## Memory-stories and narrative analysis

The basis of this way of interpreting memory-stories comes from research indicating that 'the experience of some emotions is associated with the increased recall of emotionally congruent memories' (Conway 1990, p.94). This may be explained by reference to context effect, where the mood of the present recalls an analogous mood in the past which accompanied the encoding of a particular memory. It is therefore possible 'that the experience of an emotion will activate certain knowledge structures in memory and these knowledge structures may have been employed on previous occasions when a congruent mood was experienced and an event encoded into memory' (Conway 1990, p.94). This, then, formed a cognitive model for explaining the selection bias of memories. And it was this model which Laura used in her own work and which I came to use in my evaluation, as a way of understanding the function of memory-stories recounted by people with dementia.

But other explanations in terms of function served could also be true. For memory could also be seen (as it was most famously by Proust) as that which serves to construct, or reconstruct, our sense of identity – the narrative of self. As Oliver Sacks wrote:

> If we wish to know about a man, we ask 'What is his story?' – for each of us is a biography, a story. Each of us is a singular narrative, which is constructed continually, unconsciously, by, through, and in us – through our perceptions, our feelings, our thoughts, our actions; and not least our discourse, our spoken narrations ... To be ourselves we must have ourselves – possess, if need be, repossess, our life-stories. We must 'recollect' ourselves, recollect the inner drama, the narrative of ourselves. A man needs such a narrative, a continuous inner narrative, to maintain his identity, his self. (Sacks 1985, p.105)

Both of these models – the cognitive and the phenomenological – could be fruitful in attempting to understand the world of the elderly person with dementia. Understanding the process of communication was the key to understanding the content of the message. Thus elderly clients' memory-stories of events long past were interpreted as metaphors of present feelings. I tried to follow Oliver Sacks's advice:

> The brain's record of everything … must be iconic. This is the final form of the brain's record, even though the preliminary form may be computational or programmatic. The final form of cerebral representation must be, or allow, 'art' – the artful scenery and melody of experience and action. By the same token, if the brain's representations are damaged or destroyed … their reconstitution demands a double approach – an attempting to reconstruct damaged programs and systems … or a direct approach at the level of inner melodies and scenes. (Sacks 1985, p.141)

It was this second 'direct' approach that I used in first allowing the client respondents to 'sing their own song' as far as possible in the interview situation, and then trying to read the score, as it were, not only to pick out the major themes, but to follow the analogies and metaphors which they used to orchestrate them. Psychoanalysis long ago pointed out how everyone's mental operations proceeded in this way. During the process of writing up my research I discovered the process operating in my own subconscious. I was fascinated to see that in 'anonymising' a particular transcription by rechristening the respondent, I thought that I had plucked the name 'Samuel' at random 'out of the air'. However, as I reread it, it struck me immediately that the memory-story which 'Samuel' recounted no less than three times began with how, as a young lad, he had been lying in bed at night when he heard the sound of someone calling. In rechristening him 'Samuel' I had clearly been harking back to the scriptural story of the boy Samuel.

Such, then, are our natural thought-paths. It made sense to me to follow them in trying to comprehend meaning through symbol, story and metaphor in the discourse of elderly people with dementia. Instead of stopping at the stumbling block of amnesia and dysphasia, I tried to cultivate the language of affect. This is not a new idea, and psychology and psychotherapy are not the only disciplines to use the interpretation of stories to understand meaning. A narrative approach has been used, for example, by ethnography and sociology. For stories tell us about their narrators. They also tell us about ourselves, and about the nature of the communication (or the lack of it) between us. And so it seemed appropriate to adopt a (very) quasi-ethnographic approach to the study of individual client transcripts. That is, I sought to use an understanding of narrative to interpret the communication of one social group (people with dementia) in a way that was meaningful to another (people without dementia).

## How to do it

So much for the theory. But what about the actual practice? Before I could interview any of the clients (or, indeed, their family carers) I had to have permission from the ethics committee of the (then) District Health Authority. This meant that I had to prepare a detailed protocol for submission. Although this proved a time-intensive exercise, I actually found it extremely valuable in that it not only forced an exploration of the wider ethical ramifications of the research methods, but also it had practical value in making me think through many down-to-earth issues and potential problems ahead of time. This greatly increased my confidence as I encountered the practicalities of actual interviewing for the first time. While the benefit to clients (or patients) is what is rightly uppermost in our minds when we think about ethics committees, it is important to recognise just how helpful they can be, especially to new and inexperienced researchers. I should like to put my own gratitude on record.

In the invitation letter to each family carer, which explained the nature and purpose of the evaluation and how I was carrying it out, I also explained that I would be hoping to engage their relative at Green House in a short interview to ascertain their feelings about it. In the event only two family carers said that they did not want either themselves or their relative to be involved. The majority were pleased to be consulted. Rather than writing to clients I spent a lot of time at Green House, getting to know people and hoping that they would get to feel a sense of familiarity with me. I was interested to find that, despite short-term memory loss, clients in the day-hospital often greeted me with a warm smile of recognition, an invitation to sit down and have a cup of tea, and solicitous inquiries after my well-being – before asking my name! I hoped that there were residual emotional memories laid down, and eventually I felt able to begin asking people if I could interview them. No one refused. At this point both I and the person to be interviewed would sign an agreement of confidentiality, the format for which had first been passed by the ethics committee.

Laura's method involved tape-recording the interview. Then a verbatim transcription was made from the recording. She then applied discourse analysis to the transcript. Accordingly I purchased for the study a small tape-recorder with a tiny, very sensitive lapel microphone. The expense was more than compensated for by the peace of mind of knowing that it would be possible to hear every word. Given the inevitable problems of muttering, whispering, coughing, fidgeting, and 'noises off', I was subsequently very glad that I had invested in sensitive and reliable equipment. It enabled me to concentrate on the interview itself, without having to worry unduly about the technical side of things. I was also very lucky in finding an experienced transcriber. Not only her accuracy but also her speed were particularly helpful to me, because it meant that I could read over each interview soon after it was done, while my memory of it was still fresh. It also meant that I could learn from my mistakes, and apply that learning to the next interview.

## My experience

Before the Green House evaluation I had had no experience of interviewing at all. I began by interviewing staff, managers and family carers. So by the time I came to interviewing the clients I had already gained considerable experience in interviewing people, and the surprises and challenges which it can present. Listening at length and in depth to very stressed or very vulnerable people talking about difficult and painful experiences is taxing for the interviewer at both the intellectual and the emotional level. I had read very extensively around the subject of research interviewing in general at the outset of the data-gathering. There were two books I found especially helpful. The first was Jack Douglas's book *Creative Interviewing*, which is both the most memorable and the most humorous text on depth inter- viewing on delicate subject matter (Douglas 1985). I found his concepts of the interviewer as 'the handmaiden,' the respondent as 'the goddess', and the interview situation as 'the lifeboat' springing vividly to mind in moments of internal questioning during many of my interviews with people with – or without – dementia. The second book was Elliot Mishler's *Research Interviewing* (1986), with its explo- ration of the 'joint construction of meaning' – that is, of the interview as the joint product of two people, rather than one person's interro- gation of another. It was a reminder to include myself – who I was, why I was there, what I brought to the situation – in my interpreta- tion of the interview.

Although my interviews with the staff and managers of Green House, as well as the interviews with family carers, lasted at least one or two hours, all interviews with clients of the service lasted only about twenty minutes to half-an-hour. I found this to be a reasonable limit, beyond which I felt that both parties' energy flagged. I focused on just one question: 'What is it like for you here at Green House?' Sometimes, with some clients, we were able to progress to more specific matters, but this was relatively rare. I had learned from Laura that my job as interviewer was to ask my question and then support the person I was interviewing through their own train of thought – even if I could not initially understand the relevance of what they said. That often had to wait for the transcript to illuminate it.

I found that I needed to be very patient, often waiting up to thirty seconds or even a minute, while someone slowly processed what they were trying to express and formulated it into a sentence. I also had to help support them through their search for words. It was a great art to sit quietly and patiently, with absolutely no appearance of hurry or concern, but every appearance of interest and appreciation – while the person might look as if they had forgotten what they were saying.

Amazingly I discovered that they usually *did* continue with the same train of thought after such long pauses. On these occasions it felt like conducting an interview in slow motion. Conversely, I found that it was helpful to support the more loquacious person by reflecting back gently from time to time what had just been said, thereby encouraging continuation of that train of thought. And from time to time during the course of an interview it was appropriate to summarise and reflect back what I had understood from what had been said. I found this to be a very productive way of eliciting further exposition and clarification.

Finally, like so many people in all kinds of interviews, elderly people with dementia would often respond expansively to the ending of an interview, to being thanked for their time and effort, and to appreciation of their valuable personal contribution. This very often led into further and even more rewarding exposition. 'In my end is my beginning!' In fact, I found that elderly people with dementia often needed just that reassurance of being made to feel valued and valuable. They also often needed validation of their feelings and opinions. This was where so-called 'reality orientation' could miss the point. Rather than trying to insist that they appreciated 'our' reality, it was surely more important that we learned to appreciate theirs. A confused elderly person who was grieving for someone long dead, with feelings of loss (perhaps never worked through at the time) that surfaced freshly painful, needed to have their sense of bereavement recognised and their feelings validated. It only increased confusion and lowered self-esteem to point out to them that this was 1992 and that that person had died thirty years ago.

The ethics committee protocol had stated my willingness to curtail any interview in which undue distress was evident in the respondent. In the event this did not happen. People often wept as they recounted certain experiences and feelings. I would continue to listen intently, expressing sympathy for them the while. The result was always that they seemed to 'move through' the deeper waters and then climb out on the other shore. By the end of the interview they always seemed to feel much better. I always took care after the interview ('on the way to the door', so to speak) to find a congenial and positive or sometimes humorous subject of conversation, so that the experience came to a pleasant conclusion. I was aware, however, that this did as much for me as for my respondents.

The first day's interviews (three in number) provided the first surprise. I had decided to begin by interviewing clients in the day-hospital, since, given that they were relatively less impaired, they would probably be more straightforward to interview. It was quite a shock to discover just how 'unproblematic' they actually were. Having arrived freshly armed with new techniques for interviewing confused elderly people, I was confused myself to find that the clients appeared not to be so! Having graciously granted the request for an interview, that is evidently exactly what they were expecting. Each client answered the initial questions about how it felt for them coming to Green House with seeming ease, and then waited politely for the next question. I had to do some quick thinking at this stage, and decided that I should proceed in the manner that the respondents were obviously expecting. I therefore continued to ask various questions about food, transport, activities, choices, and so on.

When this happened during the first interview I was surprised. When the next two interviews were the same I became decidedly uncomfortable and wondered if, in fact, their diagnoses were correct, or if everything I thought I knew about dementia was incorrect. In fact, I had merely discovered the enormous range of variation in ability/disability that 'dementia' covers. I had thought that all elderly people with dementia were alike. I had mentally homogenised 'them', falling into the trap of thinking not in terms of individual human beings, but in categories: not of people, but of patients. This was an important and salutary lesson at the outset – all the more so given what many of their interviews were to reveal.

As these interviews continued it became clear how unpredictable each respondent could be, and how different one from another. Some interviews could be conducted on a 'normal' question-and-answer basis, some were facilitated monologues, some were philosophical discussions, some were the rehearsal of issues and memories that the respondent needed to 'work through' or sort out to their own satis-faction. Some were extremely difficult, requiring the acceptance of the respondent's pace and style. This could mean a 'slow-motion' interview, with long pauses between responses, during which it was critical to maintain a completely patient, interested and supportive stance, as the client wrestled with dysphasia, and to judge correctly the need (or not) for further prompting or reminders. 'You must think I'm awfully stupid', the respondent might say defensively. It was important to demonstrate the opposite by volunteering solidarity in face of the common problem of 'TOTs' – tip-of-the-tongue word searches – which is an infuriation that everyone has to deal with at times. 'I often can't find the word either', had to be indicated without seeming patronising.

Imagination and intuition were crucial ingredients in semi- or unstructured interviewing, and particularly so in these client inter-views. It was necessary to enter into the respondent's world to try to capture the essence of what they were trying to communicate (Sutton and Hopkins 1994). Their past experience or areas of expertise could often be the key to their perspective. The mathematician or the administrator, the craftsman or the salesman, the parent or the child – all surfaced during these interviews to share their perspectives on Green House. It was important to understand the vantage point (and the language that belonged to it) in order to understand the view. The composer Pauline Oliveros advised: 'Offer your experience as your truth' (Le Guin 1989). It was their experience, their truth, that the clients of Green House had to offer to those with the commitment, patience and imagination to listen.

Another way in which my client respondents were like so many of the respondents in the other groups was the way they appeared to enjoy the experience. People with and without dementia value the opportunity of being consulted, and all the more so when it is in an 'interview' format. Here the microphone and recorder, which had initially worried me, proved unexpectedly useful. Their purpose would be explained to the interviewee with dementia as being an adjunct to my memory – a reminder of what I did not want to forget. This they instantly appreciated, given their own memory problems, and it helped establish equality between us. I would often add (while attaching the microphone to their clothing): 'It's like the BBC, isn't it?!' This always produced a smile, which I came to realise was the sign of a real inward gratification – a feeling of self-importance. Respondents would straighten their shoulders a little, or clear their throat. Any initial nervousness very soon disappeared, but appeared in any case to be more than compensated for by the boost to self-esteem that the situation (symbolised by the technical apparatus) had conferred.

I was gladdened afterwards to feel that I had been able to give something immediate back to them in return for their trouble, since for several of them the interview represented a very real effort. These people were obviously a little drained at the end of fifteen or twenty minutes. Nevertheless, it was reassuring that they all felt able to indicate this (always politely) so that the duration as well as the content of the interview was in their hands. One or two clients apparently enjoyed their interviews so much that whenever they saw me arrive thereafter they would make a bee-line for me with evident pleasurable expectancy! Although short-term memory impairment would appear to render it unlikely that they would remember either me or the interview, somehow an 'emotional memory' (perhaps of having been listened to) seemed to remain, and I could have conducted several interviews apiece with these respondents. In the interests of equality across groups, however, I resisted the temptation!

## Analysis: content, discourse and narrative

When it came to analysing the transcripts of these interviews I concentrated on interpretating the latent meanings, the meanings that lay behind the words said, for I followed Laura Sutton's hypothesis that elderly people with dementia use the language of long-term episodic memories as metaphors and analogies of present feelings (Sutton 1993). So within an overall discourse analysis approach to access latent meanings, I focused in particular on these narratives.

What do I mean by a discourse analysis approach? Discourse analysis as a method covers quite a variety of techniques, and its practitioners come from a variety of disciplines. A broad definition of it would be that it is a way of analysing language (be that in speech or text), developed by scholars of literature, psychology, sociology and other disciplines, in an attempt to uncover the meanings and interpretations through which speakers construct their experience of reality. It proceeds from a view that in addition to the manifest, explicit content of what is said (or written) there is also latent, implicit content which needs to be brought to the surface so that we can understand the way in which people see their world.

The importance of understanding how people see their world is rooted in the social constructionist perspective, which represents a radical move away from the concept of an objective reality 'out there' which ever-increasing accuracy of observation and measurement will reveal, and towards the concept of a multiplicity of subjective perspectives in which 'reality' is constructed in and through the mind of the beholder. So social constructionism is the epistemological position, and discourse analysis its tool.

For our purposes here the study of signs (semiotics) and the study of interpretation (hermeneutics) provide useful conceptualisations. In the semiotics of de Saussure (1974), and subsequently Barthes (1964), a sign may be divided into two parts: the signifier (a word or symbol) and the signified (a meaning). Language therefore is the code of signifiers on which discourse draws to express given meanings. A signifier may also have a secondary level of signification whereby a range of further meanings may become attached to it. For example, to talk of 'Westminster' is not only to refer to a part of London, but is also synonymous with power, British political life, a system of government. Another way of expressing this is to distinguish within the potentially multiple meanings of words between 'denotative' and 'connotative', or explicit and implicit meanings. In hermeneutics Paul

Ricoeur (1976) refers to this as 'surplus of meaning'. By this he means that within our discourse there may be several distinct yet simultaneous levels of communication occurring, including the 'poetic' levels of metaphor and symbol. He concludes that it is this unique combination of explicit and implicit meanings which is the essential characteristic of metaphor (Ricoeur 1976). If we use radio broadcasting as an analogy for metaphor, then the word 'Westminster' with its explicit meaning (a part of London) is like the carrier wave, which also carries the signal for 'the government', 'the mother of parliaments,' a particular system of democratic representation.

Discourse analysis is a methodology which is contested by those who hold an essentialist view of reality as objective, 'really there', and therefore susceptible to empirical positivist investigation. It is sometimes even perceived as inherently destructive of the discipline which harbours it – a sort of cuckoo in the nest. However, the proponents of discourse analysis as a tool of psychological investigation frame it as being precisely appropriate to social psychology, whose subject matter is human interrelating:

> because social psychologists essentially study themselves they cannot achieve the level of objectivity of, say, a chemist studying a compound or a geographer studying a landform. Since complete objectivity is unattainable, scientific methods, particularly experimental ones, are simply inappropriate for social psychology. (Hogg and Vaughan 1995)

When I say that I took a discourse analysis *approach* I mean that I did not investigate the details of extended vowels, the exact timing of gaps and pauses, audible intakes of breath, etc. as a full discourse analysis would require. Instead I focused on the two key concepts of *context* and *function*. I paid attention, for example, to the *context* in which a given narrative (or opinion or observation) occurred in the interview. What had we been talking about just beforehand, which the interviewee had used as a take-off point for his or her memory-story? And what were the salient features of the literal context in which the story was being told – for example, what was going on in the day-room at that time? Here, of course, I needed to rely on my field notes, although some audible features of the environment were actually recorded (and therefore transcribed). I also paid attention to the *function* which the story (or opinion or observation) seemed to achieve, or designed to achieve. What turn did the conversation take from there? What was the very next thing the interviewee said? With regard to the memory-stories in particular I kept asking the questions: 'Why this particular story at this particular point in the conversation, in this particular place? And how does it tie in with the rest of what this particular person is telling me?'

Why did I choose this method? I could give two reasons. The first is that I was taking a phenomenological approach to my evaluation of Green House, trying to capture its multi-dimensionality. I had eschewed the model of 'one reality' at the outset. But the second reason was that I favoured discourse analysis as an approach which acknowledges the individual as an agent of meaning. Given that I had accorded the respondents from the other three stakeholder groups that same status, I thought it only appropriate to employ a method which would do the same for the elderly clients with dementia. In other words, I tried to give all interviewees equivalent status as agents of meaning, not by using the same method for everybody, but rather by using methods that were appropriate for different types of respondents.

## Practical implications

Clearly it is not feasible to use this method of first recording interviews, then transcribing them and analysing the transcripts, on a regular basis. While it constitutes an invaluable tool for exploring the concerns and viewpoints of individual elderly clients with dementia, especially when trying to evaluate or audit a service, it does, nevertheless, represent a very considerable investment of time and effort. On the other hand, it is perhaps only a proper redressing of the balance that we should expend such time and effort on ascertaining the point of view of our elderly clients with dementia, after ignoring them so consistently, and with such terrible effect, for so long. We owe them at least our best listening time, and 'the imagination of our hearts' in seeking to understand them.

And that, I believe, is the practical lesson to be drawn from this method. To use it is to acquire a certain 'ear'. Spending many hours listening to memory-stories, and then poring over transcripts, leads to a certain sensitivity for the metaphorical content of so much of what is said around one. I found that I learned to hear implied meanings in what people (with or without dementia) were saying, in ways which I had not before. I can best describe this as having an ear for the poetry of ordinary conversations. Michael Polanyi said that 'we know more than we can tell' (Polanyi 1966). Using this method taught me that we also tell more than we know. Reading the transcripts was like reading the text of a play – but one in which I had myself taken part.

As I reread the lines, two things happened. First, they stimulated a variety of rich images in my mind. When I read one old man's memory of women in the street during the First World War, pinning the white feather of cowardice on men of fighting age who were not in uniform (which had happened to his father), a whole scene of unpredictable threat and unreasoning prejudice was conjured up in my mind's eye. Second, these images helped (I could say forced) me to identify with the feelings they engendered. The narrator of the story of the white feathers had told me much of a rigidly gendered upbringing and outlook; surrounded by women at home and in the day-hospital, he was humiliated by his frailty and dependence, although for the most part he put on a brave and sociable face.

Realising how much, in our discourse, we give away of our feelings, our needs, and our deep concerns leads not only to greater understanding, but also to a sense of the responsibility we carry: as actors on each other's stage, and as supporters of each other's fragile identity. We do not need tape-recorders or transcribers to accept elderly people with dementia as agents of meaning, with perspectives and interpretations, or to cultivate a sensitivity to the metaphorical meanings – the 'poetic' imagery – of the memory-stories they tell, and apply this imaginatively to their present situation. Older people with dementia certainly know more than they can tell; but if we are prepared to enter the world of their imagery with them they can tell us more than they – or we – know.

## Dementia Care Mapping

Not all of the clients at Green House were able to be interviewed, since for some of them speech had become all but impossible. This was, however, a matter of degree, and I therefore found it possible to interview many clients with considerable speech impairment. Nevertheless it seemed unfair to accept only those client perceptions of Green House that could be verbally expressed, recorded and transcribed. And so I needed an alternative method of gaining some insight into clients' experience of Green House – a method which was not reliant on verbal skills.

It was at this point that I was fortunate enough to be put in touch with Dr Tom Kitwood and Kathleen Bredin at Bradford University, who were developing such a method, precisely to furnish information for evaluations such as mine. It was called Dementia Care Mapping (DCM), and relied on observational data collected using time frames and activity codes to which positive or negative 'Care Values' were attached. In this way it was possible to 'map' the perceived experience of individual clients in a given group care setting. Nowadays DCM has become quite a well-known tool, and through extensive use it has evolved in sophistication beyond the original prototype which I first encountered. The tool to which I refer here is the original DCM method as it was used for the Green House evaluation. Much has been published about DCM; here I shall merely give an overview in order to show how I was able to build up the picture of clients experience as well as their views of the service.

DCM was based on a certain view of dementia and a corresponding philosophy of care. Tom Kitwood took issue with the standard paradigm of dementia as an irremediable disease of neurological deterioration, and put forward instead the idea of dementia as a process – a downward spiral involving the critical interaction of neurological impairment and a 'malignant social psychology' (Kitwood 1990):

> When self-esteem is lacking or damaged, a person is disastrously incapacitated in many ways, and easily falls into a cycle of discouragement and failure ... The quality of an individuals self-esteem has its counterpart at the neurochemical level. Each aspect of the malignant social psychology is, in some way, damaging to self-esteem, and tends to diminish personhood; that is why it merits the epithet 'malignant'. When a person has been subjected to a predominantly malignant social psychology for several years, the effects may indeed be devastating. Remarkably, the greater part of medical science research on dementia seems to overlook this altogether. (Kitwood 1990)

The DCM method therefore coded such episodes of 'malignant social psychology' as 'personal detractions' (PDs). These were listed in five increasing levels of severity, and were recorded in an attempt to investigate what contributed to that state of ill-being. PDs ranged from the mild (such as 'outpacing' – doing things faster than the person with dementia could cope with) through things like speaking in front of someone as if they were not present, to treating them as an object, insulting or demeaning them, and finally to cruel banishment and physical assault.

Indeed, it was this recognition of the enormous intrinsic importance of the quality and nature of interpersonal care experienced by the elderly person with dementia that underlay Tom Kitwood's sociopsychological model, and was used in DCM as the key to evaluation. That is, the care environment was evaluated in terms of the measured levels of well-being or ill-being of individual clients:

> The DCM method was developed to augment other more structural types of evaluation with a detailed assessment of what is happening at the person-to-person level of care ... [It] is based on looking for evidence of relative well-being, and assumes a rough equation, when a number of sufferers are involved: relative

> well-being = good quality care, as well as its converse: relative
> ill-being = poor quality care. (Kitwood and Bredin 1994)

Well-being in dementia was identified with four global subjective states: a sense of personal worth, of agency, of social confidence, and of hope.

Someone using DCM could track several clients at a time – usually about five. At five-minute intervals the 'mapper' would record activity codes for each client, expressing the dominant activity of importance for them during that period. For example, eating or drinking was coded 'F', walking 'K', sleeping 'N', and so on. The choice of what activity code (or 'Behaviour Category Codes' as they were called) to record in any given time frame was made within well-defined rules. For example, an 'activity', such as eating or walking, always super-seded inactivity (or 'social domain' categories) such as passive involvement with the environment, distress, or sleeping. The mapper also recorded a 'Care Value' (positive or negative) against each behaviour category code, denoting the individual client's perceived level of well-or ill-being, in accordance with well-defined frames of reference and guidelines.

From the completed raw data sheets a variety of analyses could be made. The most fundamental level of analysis was the 'Individual Care Score'. For each individual client mapped, a care score was calculated which reflected their experience of the care provided in terms of how far it had contributed to their personhood by supporting their well-being. A range of scores in the DCM manual were provided, against which each given Individual Care Score could be measured. These ranged from 'much improvement needed' through 'fair', 'good', 'very good', and 'excellent.' In this way the care provided in the environment was measured in terms of how it con-tributed to the well-being and supported the personhood of any given individual client.

These Individual Care Scores could then be aggregated and an average – or 'Group Care Score' – calculated. This provided an indicator of the general level of care provided in the facility. However, the method recognised that it was necessary to take into account the staff-to-patient ratio, and so a subsequent calculation was made, called the 'Dementia Care Quotient' (DCQ) – which stabilised the group care score against a given norm. In this way the DCQ effectively either 'penalised' for a generous staffing ratio or 'rewarded' for an inadequate one. This calculation was particularly valuable in that it increased the credibility of the method in the eyes of staff.

Two other analyses were also useful. First the 'Behaviour Category Profile' showed the prevalence of different types of activity – or lack of them – both for individual clients and in the environment in general. For example, a traditional, soporific long-stay ward is often found to have a 'BCN' profile, where 'B' corresponds to 'just looking around', 'C' to apathy and withdrawal, and 'N' to sleep. Similarly it was possible to construct a Care Value Profile for both individuals and the environment in general. The latter was particularly instructive since it showed an evaluation of the care environment in terms of overall levels of well-being and ill-being. Using this analysis it was possible to track over time what changes did, or did not, occur in these levels.

These analyses were completed as quickly as possible so that the staff on duty could be given immediate feedback. The Behaviour Category Codes (BCCs) refer to a variety of interactional contexts (including absence of interaction, where 'C', for example, is the code for 'apathy and withdrawal'), within which the well-being or ill-being of an individual with dementia is being measured. For example, how positive or negative an experience of care is eating and drinking (F) for a given client? Is it 'highly therapeutic' (in which case it is given a care value of +5)? Or does it show 'slight ill-being' (in which case it is given a care value of −1)? And above all what were the facilitating factors? Why was, for instance, a meal such a good experience, or why did it lead to withdrawal or restlessness? This is where the developmental ethos came into play, as staff were encouraged, on feedback of these results, to explore strategies which would increase the well-being of that client, for example, at meal-times.

The DCM method was not unproblematic. To begin with, it was not value-free. Indeed, Tom and Kathy were explicit in their recognition of the fact that it was deliberately value-laden. Its explicit purpose was 'developmental evaluation'. That is, it was designed to evaluate care in such a way as to clarify the directions required for positive changes – both at the individual and whole-environment levels. In fact, it was precisely this developmental potential which was subsequently to be used in Green House. Here it is important to say that both the staff of Green House (who were always given immediate feedback) and I as evaluator recognised that the findings from data gathered using the DCM method proceeded from a clear value perspective.

Another possible criticism was that DCM was only used in group settings, since it would be not only intrusive, but also create artificiality, to follow individual clients and care-givers into private and intimate settings such as bathrooms and bedrooms. It was assumed that the experience of care would not be that different in those settings, since the care-givers and clients are the same people in both settings and, most importantly, care staff could not demonstrate skills which they did not possess. This brings us to the problem of most observational methods, that is the so-called 'Hawthorne effect': that the very fact of being observed alters people's behaviour. However, it was rare for any of the clients to display such a change, and with regard to the staff, at best it meant that the presence of an observer had raised the level of care for clients and perhaps made staff more aware of what they were capable of achieving. This was one reason why it was very important to feed back to the staff involved as soon as possible what care mapping had indicated of clients' experience, since this could act as positive reinforcement.

The Care Values themselves represented a problem for the mathematical purist. For they were qualitatively different entities, and not points on a continuous scale. Hence +5 and +3 referred to two different kinds of experience (albeit both positive). Theoretically it would be possible to use not numbers but words: for example, they could be 'apples' and 'oranges'. Since the Care Values are added together in order to be divided by the time frames, so that an Individual Care Score can be calculated for each client 'mapped', the criticism runs that different things were being added together to give a single result. While this was true, there was a pragmatic logic in using numbers for the Care Values, since what was being measured was the 'positiveness' or 'negativeness' of a given experience for a given individual client. Intuitively, then, we respond to greater or smaller numbers as representing the increase or decrease in well-being engendered by the experience.

Similarly, the objective of the method as originally invented was to stimulate positive changes in care. So a 'scoring' system certainly generated that inner competitiveness which makes us always want to see higher scores. However, when it came to analysing the data using Care Value Profiles, the significance of the results were tested statistically using chi-squared. This was in recognition of the fact that the Care Values actually represent non-scaleable data. (While parametric tests could be more precise, they should only be applied to genuinely scaleable data – which Care Values are not.)

As this method was at that time still unpublished, I was very fortunate in being able to make contact with its authors. I was even more fortunate in that they agreed to come to teach me the method, and help with the initial observations, actually at Green House, so that between the three of us we could track simultaneously all the clients in either the day-hospital or the in-patient unit. After Tom and Kathy went back to Bradford I used to send them the results of my own 'mapping' on an ad hoc basis for checking and correction.

Before Tom and Kathy arrived I prepared the ground by discussing the method fully with as many as possible of the Green House staff. I discussed it in separate groups, first with qualified and then with unqualified staff. Their enthusiasm and the warm welcome they gave to the whole idea were impressive. This was not only a tribute to their professionalism and humanitarian values, but it also showed how hungry staff in this field of care were for feedback on how their patients actually experienced the care delivered. For these were clients with whom they often found communication difficult, and so it was demotivating for them to do work that was both physically and emotionally demanding with very little feedback or reinforcement. It was precisely this feedback which they were anxious to have. As I had already interviewed most of them individually by that time, the idea of my sitting in the care environment with pad and pencil did not seem as strange or as potentially threatening as it might otherwise have done.

Tom and Kathy were welcomed also, not only as pioneering researchers in the field, but as sources of information. This constituted an illuminating indication of the need for clinical psychological input in care environments for people with dementia. The staff used the opportunity to question and discuss a variety of concerns with them. It was a crucial part of the DCM method to work cooperatively with staff, and not as 'time-and-motion-men' come to evaluate their performance. What we were trying to evaluate, after all, was the clients' experience, and only indirectly the practice of care staff. However, feedback sessions during the handovers at the end of each shift were obviously carefully attended to, because subsequently we used to notice certain changes in practice. Despite the possible criticisms of it, therefore, I was particularly pleased to have found a research method that made the benefits of the evaluation immediately available to those actually delivering care.

## A result of the method

In fact, the use of this particular research method had important consequences, not only for Green House, but for the organisation (a mental health care trust) to which it belonged. For the discovery of the consciousness-raising, attitude-changing properties of 'mapping' prompted the organisation to set up a pilot project to look at its usefulness as a quality tool. The necessary funding was found from regional clinical audit monies.

Later on, in Chapter Seven, we shall look at what happened when awareness of clients' daily experience of life in the care environment was facilitated by the DCM project. Here it is sufficient to say that in addition to Green House, staff from four other dementia care facilities took part in this project. They were drawn from all disciplines: nurses, occupational therapists, domestic staff, porters, a consultant, clinical managers, senior managers (including the Trust's Chief Executive and the Chair of the purchasing Health Commission), clinical psychologists, and two family carers. They were all trained in the method by Tom, and as project manager I was able to provide ongoing support as each one mapped in their own ward and fed back immediately at the end of their mapping shift to their colleagues in staff handover, adapting care plans as necessary. People often found this process of illumination emotionally challenging, as they saw with great clarity the emptiness, sadness and frustration which filled so much of their clients' time. Nevertheless the use of DCM was accepted with enthusiasm, and a culture of openness to feedback and the beginnings of a person-centred approach to care were created. The success of the project encouraged other Trusts to train their staff in the method too.

The Green House staff were remarkable in their particular ownership of the method. The majority of them remembered how their unit had been part of the final polishing of the method, during Tom and Kathy's visit. This, together with the appointment of an outstanding new ward manager (who quickly qualified as an 'advanced' mapper), led Green House to embrace the method enthusiastically as a tool for staff training, for audit, and for generating better information to make a reality of the process of assessing client needs.

## Practical implications

From the whole experience of using DCM as an evaluative tool I would draw three practical conclusions. Clearly the full implementation of a DCM evaluation – let alone an ongoing, large-scale training project – does not come without a cost, and for a variety of reasons may not always be practicable. There are, however, practical insights to be learned from it. First, what those of us who have used DCM have learned is the very simple lesson that we need to trust the ordinary, everyday, intuitive skills which we use to read the body language, emotional state, and abilities and disabilities of our fellow human beings. These are not special skills; we all possess them, and we all use them all the time. In fact, it would not be possible to learn to use DCM if we did not have these skills. It is just that when we are dealing with elderly people with dementia we do not apply them as we would normally. An old man sits slumped forward in his chair with his head in his hands, staring at the floor. It is not difficult to read dejection and depression. Yet I have seen people walk past someone in this state with no recognition that he might be in deep distress. They will say that he is always like that – it is his condition. But conditions do not get depressed; people do. We can apply the normal skills of reading behaviour instead of switching them off as we enter a care environment. We can respond to the person, rather than the 'condition'.

The second practical implication to which I would draw attention is from the DCM project as a whole, when all those who had contact with elderly clients with dementia were offered not only the training but also the opportunity to use the method. That is, they would spend a whole shift, on a regular basis, just observing in detail the lives of their clients as they unfolded before them. The value of this to all staff was inestimable. For they recognised that observation is as much a part of the job of delivering care as activity, and that people can learn and gain important practical insight into what can make a difference to the experience of their clients if they are given that opportunity to exercise their observational skills. In the last chapter I shall consider the costs of care. Here I would just say that activity unsupported by observation can lead to much wasted time and effort – and wasted time and effort is a cost.

Finally, I believe it is also true that, apart from observation, it is valuable to spend time just sitting, just 'being', alongside elderly clients with dementia. Over the years I have spent many hundreds of hours, sitting 'mapping' in a variety of care environments. When I first started with Tom and Kathy I felt uncomfortable. But I learned to find a low place – a low chair, a footstool or the floor – and just to settle into being in that environment, just as my fellows in that environment were just 'being'. I remember the first time I went into a very soporific in-patient lounge in Green House and sat down to begin a whole shift's mapping. It was with great surprise that I realised how at home I felt, as one or two of my fellow sitters nodded to me. We waited for the tea-trolley together. Whether mapping or not, just spending time 'being' alongside people gives an insight into their world and their subjective reality which nothing else can. And in doing so we can offer our companionship. Sometimes that is all we have to offer, but it is no small thing.

## Conclusion

There will, of course, be other ways of accessing the perspective of elderly people with dementia on the services they use. We need to be alert to them, and to the possibilities of finding them which new experiences suggest. This is where media such as the *Journal of Dementia Care* are so useful. They spread ideas, experience and good practice – thereby stimulating new possibilities. But this is precisely the point: new methods of understanding will only grow from our experiences of using existing ones. Using existing methods will inevitably have its effect upon our attitudes to, and our relationships with, elderly people with dementia. It is from these changing, evolving attitudes and relationships that new ways of understanding and communicating will grow in their turn. It is an ongoing, iterative process. But it will not happen unless we begin to use the tools and the abilities that we have.

# CHAPTER 3

# The story of Green House

*The ways in which services for people with dementia are planned and brought into being show us our dedication to providing the best we can, the pitfalls of implementation, and who is and is not listened to in the process.*

Green House had memory-stories of its own. As we move on from discussing ways of listening, I want to stop along the way, and set the scene for what is to follow: the exploration of what these methods actually furnished. So in this chapter we shall look at how Green House came into being. It is a story set in interesting times, a story of commitment to an ideal of providing care in the community for elderly people with dementia. It is a story of how a variety of caring and enlightened people strove to create the best possible facility for their clients against a background of shifting requirements, massive organisational change at both national and local levels, and considerable local misunderstanding and opposition. It is an example of how the implementation path of rational strategic planning 'never does run smooth', and this despite so many good intentions, so much imagination and ingenuity, and often Herculean efforts. For it was also a story of misunderstanding, lack of communication, bitter disappointment, and tragedy.

No one wanted Green House to be anything other than successful; but no-one sought the views of its potential clients. Throughout this story the absence of the clients' point of view is striking. Of course, it is only remarkable if we proceed from a 'naive' assumption of 'client-centred' care. This is what professionals say they base their practice on, and around which managers say they design services. Yet the service and building design of Green House included no input from clients – other than acquiescence at the fait accompli.

It is an interesting (but surely not unique) example of the problems which can bedevil the implementation of the policy of 'community care,' and which probably lurk inherently within the capacious folds of its ill-defined and 'all-things-to-all-people' linguistic cloak. Significantly, many of those I interviewed found it difficult to define who was meant by 'the community'. Answers varied from 'everyone outside Green House' through 'Joe Public – you and I' to 'everyone in the British Isles'! However, regardless of how 'community' was defined, in seeking to provide (or in this particular instance, 'reprovide') a locally-based service for elderly people with dementia, the Health Service found itself (by the admission of its own staff and managers) in direct collision with local opinion. Constrained by limited resources while endeavouring to uphold faithfully the spirit of the community care policy, managers were unable to persuade the local population of the benefit to 'the community' of their proposals. While the arguments raged between health service and 'the community,' as well as between different health districts, within the health district and the unit concerned, and between the health authority and the builders, the little Green House day-hospital moved patiently around Riverford (not a large town) four times: from inauspicious beginnings in a community day centre, to a hospital, thence to lodge, much despised, within another hospital, until finally it came to rest in its own new building.

Green House, in the market town of Riverford, was planned and built under the auspices of what was then the mental health unit of the District Health Authority (DHA) (subsequently a mental health care NHS Trust). Green House was the first 'stand-alone' facility for elderly clients with dementia built by the DHA. It was part of the reprovision programme for one of the old psychiatric 'asylums'. Green House was called an 'integrated' facility in that it contained under one roof both a 13-place day-hospital and a 22-bed in-patient facility for both respite, assessment and continuing care, as well as a team base for the region's Psychiatry of Old Age community mental health team.

## The beginning of the story

The story begins as long ago as December 1983, when the DHA commissioned a 'Mental Illness Issue Group' to 'prepare a strategy for the care and treatment of the mentally ill in the Health District'. The Group's report was accepted by the Authority the following year, including their recommendations 'to provide an identifiable service for the elderly with psychiatric disorders throughout the District including the setting aside of beds for this purpose … in community homes. The ultimate aim is to lessen institutionalisation and enable Social Services and the community to help whilst keeping the patient close to relatives and friends.' This reflected the national policy of providing care 'in the community', so that people in need of services could have direct, local access to them.

The District's mental health unit had just acquired responsibility for the mental health of the population, which became a locality of the Springton Mental Health Unit. A new locality manager was recruited to organise services for it in 1986. There was a lot to do. With almost no other mental health provision, this area had been called 'a service desert' by the Mental Illness Issue Group. For the area depended virtually entirely on the neighbouring old psychiatric hospital for in-patient services, day-hospitals, and out-patient clinics. In this it shared the psychiatric hospital with three neighbouring health authorities. Following both national and regional policies of closing the former 'asylums', all three had agreed to collaborate on the closure of the psychiatric hospital. So the District's mental health unit began implementing a strategy to 'reprovide' its services, focused on the development of community mental health teams.

## Local planning for elderly people with dementia

What became Green House began as a provisional plan for a new 'Elderly Severely Mentally Infirm' (ESMI) facility in the town, permission for which was sought by the mental health unit in July 1987. This was part of their development of community mental health services in the former 'service desert' region. In September the newly-recruited sister/charge nurse for the planned facility came into post and, *faute de mieux*, was based initially with the Adult Community Mental Health Team. Her first task in creating a service for elderly clients with dementia in the area was to set up a day-hospital, which opened first on a one-day-a-week basis in a community day centre. 'A hopelessly inadequate building – dreadful! The access, the building, the transport were all dreadful!' said one member of the original staff team I interviewed.

Thus at the beginning of 1988 the day-hospital was moved into a disused ward of the by then virtually closed hospital for local people with very severe learning difficulties. Although this location was criticised by staff and carers as carrying too much stigma locally, here at least it was able to operate on a five-day-a-week basis; it was from this location that it acquired its name. The ward had been called 'Green Ward', and so the day-hospital took the name of 'Green Day Hospital'. Eventually its new, purpose-built facility was called 'Green House'.

Initially Springton DHA had been hoping to purchase one hospital site in the region and develop the embryonic new service from there. This proved impossible, since a financial arrangement agreeable to both health authorities involved could not be reached. The next option they explored was yet another Riverford hospital: St John's, a hospital for the elderly ('geriatrics'), which was much beloved by the local population who had raised considerable sums of money to provide extra equipment for it. It was at this time that a project team to design the new facility began to meet. It included the locality manager, the newly-recruited consultant in Old Age Psychiatry, and the new sister/charge nurse, as well as other clinical staff and members of the Capital and Estates Department charged with overseeing the project. The design for the new facility, therefore, began life as a design for redevelopment of the St John's hospital site. One of the staff involved later pointed out that this had led to much waste of their time in designing for a site which was ultimately rejected. For it was soon decided that it would have to close, and the new dementia care unit would have to be based at yet another local hospital site: the Riverford Infirmary.

This was a formative moment regarding the way the local community viewed Green House. I should point out that the DHA was unusual nationally in supporting the maintenance of community hospitals. In fact, there were to be 12 small community hospitals based in small market towns across Springton Health District, in addition to the large District General Hospital in Springton itself. But clearly only one hospital per town could be justified. So in Riverford this meant a choice between St John's and the Riverford Infirmary. The Health Authority therefore decided to close St John's and to concentrate all community services on the Infirmary site, since this already contained a small casualty department, together with X-ray, physiotherapy and out-patient services. It was also conveniently adjacent to the GP Health Centre, whose doctors provided on-call support. And so the proposed new dementia care unit would also have to be on the Infirmary site. One senior manager, in a delicate understatement, described this crucial decision as 'politically sensitive'.

Among the population of Riverford this proved an extremely unpopular decision. Local devotion to St John's and alarm at its closure led to such discontent that a public meeting was called by senior managers of the Health Authority in an attempt to explain their reasoning: that they were trying to provide the maximum in terms of local health services for the population by concentrating resources on the one most logical site. However, local feeling was barely assuaged, and found a new outlet when the proposed new site beside the Infirmary for the unit for dementia clients proved inadequate to accommodate the facility as planned without the additional acquisition of land owned by the Town Council.

Thus began the convoluted and acrimonious saga of the council 'potting shed'. Aerial photographs of the Infirmary site identified that the size and shape of the proposed building and its surrounds could be accommodated between the hospital and the GP Health Centre if an allotment beside the municipal park could be used. Bearing in mind local opposition to the closure of St John's, local councillors refused obdurately to sell this land to the Health Authority, reiterating instead the local view that the beloved St John's should be kept open, and could be used instead. Matters reached the point where the option of compulsory purchase was under serious consideration. Fortunately a change of mayor led to more reasonable negotiations resuming. And equally fortunately an elderly house-holder whose property adjoined the park decided that his garden was too big for him to cultivate, and agreed to sell a parcel of his land (an orchard) to the Health Authority on which they could 'reprovide' the greenhouse for the municipal gardeners. Hence the reprovision of the old psychiatric hospital came to include also reprovision of the municipal potting shed! One manager who had been closely involved remarked that the potting shed 'turned into a mini Kew Gardens! Quite over the top! I spent more time on this than the rest of the scheme put together! It cost £80,000 to replace! Blackmail!'

No sooner had this hurdle been negotiated than another problem arose, this time explicitly financial. In 1988 the new mental health unit manager was faced with a substantial end-of-year overspend requiring urgent action. This entailed prioritising among the planned new services in the district. With regard to its older clients, immediate savings were found by transferring assessment beds away from the psychiatric hospital and into the existing hospital service in Springton City. This caused considerable pressure on the Springton service, and it became clear that one of the priorities with regard to the reprovision programme would have to be the ESMI facility in Riverford. A sister facility in neighbouring Goughton had also been planned, but in the event this was sacrificed to financial contingencies, and the size of the Riverford facility expanded correspondingly: from 17 in-patient beds to 22. Although a day-hospital was successfully opened in Goughton, there was again much local resentment among both staff and carers, this time concerning the cancellation of their own in-patient facility. In particular this led to a problem with respite care, since day-hospital clients from Goughton had to travel 13 miles to Riverford, to a facility with which they were completely unfamiliar, and their carers felt correspondingly cut off.

Therefore even the planning and initial design stages of Green House were fraught with difficulties, disagreements, acrimony, disappointment and resentment. In particular, both the Riverford and Goughton communities were (albeit for different reasons) alienated from and antipathetic towards the new unit.

## The project team plans the building

The project team grew as it came to include a variety of clinicians and also the relevant support services' managers or their representatives. Indeed there was a determined and democratic commitment to include as many people as possible to be involved with the new unit, so that the architect (who also attended) could benefit from a variety of insights. However, to some of the participants the meetings often seemed to include too many people and to be too large. This was one reason given for the team's failure to reach consensus over certain crucial features. For example, the whole question of single occupancy bedrooms was one that bitterly divided the project team. The lines of division appeared for the most part between clinical staff (who favoured single occupancy) and Capital and Estates staff (who were trained to follow traditional Department of Health guidelines and procedures). The disagreement was eventually carried to the office of the Director of Public Health for arbitration, resulting in a compromise decision for some single rooms and some multiple occupancy. As usual in such cases, this compromise satisfied neither party – both stating subsequently that they wished they had been more forceful and carried the day.

This had two consequences. First, the architect evidently received mixed messages from the project team. Although he attended many of the meetings, the design of the finished building was adjudged by most respondents to be less than satisfactory, and to bear the hallmarks of a building designed by a committee. For example, while the day-hospital facility was pleasant and domestic in scale, the in-patient lounge was large, draughty and barn-like as a result of its high ceiling. Nor had any consideration been given to the need for a separate day-hospital entrance to obviate the need for day-hospital clients traipsing through the 'home' of the in-patient clients. The fact that all clients might not wish to have meals together led to the use of a walk-through area as a separate dining-room for the in-patient unit, which was very cramped. The dirty utility room (where bed-pans were emptied) led immediately off the living-room. In all these ways and more it was evident that the project team had failed to agree among themselves on clear guidelines for what was needed, or to work insightfully with the architect to monitor that their proposals were in fact being incorporated into the building in the way they intended.

Second, the District Health Authority became concerned that, with other similar new facilities on the strategic planning horizon, such design issues might recur to plague the decision-making processes of other teams. Consequently the District General Manager commissioned a research paper on the key issues for ESMI units, which I was asked to produce under the supervision of the Director of Public Health. This was my first introduction to the field of dementia care.

The project team faced a problem when the original project manager left the Health District to work elsewhere, while retaining his role at a distance. The immediate oversight of the project was turned over to another manager, who joined the team at the end of 1989, just when the Health Authority became concerned about the time-scale for completing the new service, aware that March 1991 was to be the date for final closure of the old psychiatric hospital. 'Fast track solutions were the order of the day,' said one manager.

Now it became clear to all concerned that management action at all levels was needed to win the race against time that this closure represented. The Mental Illness Issue Group had been re-convened as a result of a Community Health Council report (March 1989) which had identified major problems with the implementation of their original strategy. The new Issue Group Report (September 1989) said: 'A difference of expectations exists between top managers and staff, and it would be of assistance if a clear statement was produced making it quite explicit that the relocation of [the old psychiatric] Hospital patients is a reprovision of services, and not a new service.' Now the district, unit and locality reprovision groups met on a regular basis and established cross-membership of key players with, as one manager said, the District 'firmly in the driving-seat'!

Thereafter the project team's deliberations took place against a background of great haste and bustle. 'Local teams were staggered by the vigour of the top-down approach to planning decisions that were made by people that they never saw or met,' one of those involved wrote of this period. So to over-large meetings, internal divisions, and the removal to a distance of the original project manager (whose functions were devolved onto someone hitherto uninvolved in the project), was now added 'top-down' urgency and drive.

## The building of Green House

By Christmas Eve 1989 the contractors for the building had been selected. Because of the size of the project they were chosen by the Regional (rather than the District) Health Authority. Subsequently this was seen as a mistake. With hindsight the District Estates Department felt that it would have been wiser for them to have selected the contractor, and to have done so on the clarity of their proposed process. Nevertheless, in January 1990 the first holes were sunk for the foundations. A ten-month contract period had been imposed, but again with hindsight this was seen to have been too short. Fifteen to twenty months would have been normal, but due to the increased urgency for reproviding the closing old psychiatric hospital service the contract period (calculated on the basis of wishful thinking rather than realism) was reduced. So the ground was laid for the central tragedy in the building of Green House, by a combination of working with an unknown contractor, and well-intentioned scheduling to unrealistic timescales.

By spring of 1990 it was already clear that the contract was falling behind schedule. Although changing the contractor was mooted, it was clear that this would delay the process even further. However, the company's headquarters became directly involved, and at the same time the leadership of the Capital and Estates Department also changed. There was concern at the four-week delay – 'due to the weather!' although the winter had been mild. Seeing the potential for disaster, staff were instructed to increase their attendance on site to maintain a very obvious monitoring presence. Following a site inspection, in September a meeting of the project team asked the contractor for a fully-resourced programme to completion. By then it was clear that there would be slippage from the original completion date, and so discussions were opened with the neighbouring health authority ('owners' of the old psychiatric hospital) about the implications of not being able to rehouse the clients in question until a later date.

The project team made explicit representations of their great concern about the possible dangers to clients of any additional move. The third health district which had used beds at the 'psychiatric' hospital, had surpassed their own reprovision programme and withdrawn their patients (and therefore their funding) sooner than expected. This had left the health district which owned the hospital with fewer patients than planned in these final months of closure, when the hospital was in any event extremely non-cost-effective to run. They therefore felt unable, despite many emotional pleas from Springton, to keep the ward where the Springton patients were cared for open any longer.

The contractors were still four weeks behind schedule, and this slippage increased as the full implications of the highly-engineered building became clear to them. Managers I interviewed felt that this realisation had come rather late in the day, and that these implications should have been properly thought through before they started on site. With this lack of foresight and planning, then, the delay increased, and what all involved most dreaded became a necessity: the remaining ten Springton patients in the old psychiatric hospital (elderly, physically and mentally very frail) had to be moved temporarily to the already crowded wards of St Bridget's hospital in Springton, some twenty miles distant, in the bitter cold of December.

## Commissioning and moving in

If there had been haste in planning in 1989, and rising panic over the building delay in 1990, by the end of the year the efforts of the project team and every level of management reached a crescendo in their commitment to opening Green House at the very earliest possible opportunity. It was decided, therefore, that the usual twelve weeks for commissioning the building would be telescoped to an unheard-of three. This meant among other things that instead of the usual procedure for cleaning the building at the end of commissioning, the domestic team would actually clean Green House *around* the technical staff as they worked. On top of this the delivery of the furniture, equipment and supplies would take place all in one go, these things having already been collected at another site and checked ready for delivery.

It was at this point that all the staff who had been recruited for the new facility (many via re-deployment from St John's) enjoyed an induction training week. Despite the shortcomings of this training with regard to helping them actually understand both the clients and the nature of the job, it was at the time considered very successful by all concerned in establishing a good team-spirit. This was timely, for some of the new staff were sent to St Bridget's in Springton to help the over-crowded wards where their new clients were temporarily lodged. For many of them this proved quite a 'culture shock', as one staff respondent euphemistically described it.

Meanwhile the existing day-hospital team insisted on keeping the day-hospital open right up to the Friday before the Monday opening of the new building. Then, joined by several of their new 'team', in an extraordinary display of initiative and dedication they spent the weekend moving the day-hospital equipment over from the Riverford Infirmary into the new building and unwrapping and placing all the furniture and equipment appropriately around the building as it was delivered – including hanging the curtains. They were rewarded. When the day-hospital opened for business-as-usual again on the Monday morning, one elderly client looked around appreciatively and remarked: 'You've done a bit of work on the place then!'

Two days later, on Wednesday 23 January 1991, five of the ten original Springton in-patients from the old psychiatric hospital, who had been at St Bridget's in Springton, were driven over to Riverford and arrived at Green House. The staff who were there ready to welcome them remembered vividly the emotion of that moment. One nurse said that 'they looked like a band of orphans'.

The other five clients had died.

## Organisational change

Green House day-hospital opened on 21 January 1991, and the in-patient facility opened two days later, on 23 January. My involvement with it, through both the evaluation and the DCM project which grew from it, extended until 1995. Those first four years of Green House's existence took place against a background of considerable organisational change.

The result of so much determination and vision, this prototype of a 'stand-alone, integrated, locally-based ESMI unit' was not favoured by fate with an easy infancy. The major internal organisational change at Green House resulted from the long-term sick-leave and eventual resignation of the sister/charge nurse, and her replacement by a new charge nurse from outside the District. Having invested so much enthusiasm and ingenuity in the development of the service and led her exponentially expanded team through the extraordinary challenge of the super-short commissioning period, the first sister/charge nurse quickly felt her vision for enhanced standards of care undermined by inadequate staffing levels. For example, Green House's scheduled 22 beds had to be cut to 15 because the staffing levels – which had been pegged at the old psychiatric hospital levels – were deemed to be unsafe. This was just one way in which the difference between running a ward which was part of a larger hospital, and could count on all the corresponding back-up facilities, and a unit which had to be self-sufficient, became clear.

At the same time, the Mental Health Unit reorganised its geo-graphical management structure, so that the original four localities were telescoped into two. This entailed the Riverford locality being merged with Springton City, and coming under a different management team. None of the staff I later interviewed (29 in all) were happy with this, and in fact expressed very negative comments about the new management. They blamed the staffing shortages entirely on them, and interpreted the threatened overspend, for which financial stringency was the cure, as the result of management incompetence. They harked back to the former management as to a golden age of commitment and, above all, of good communication. It appeared that in amalgamating two former localities into one, management had receded a significant degree away from the front-line, and staff respondents felt both unheard and uninformed.

Staff shortages meant not only that staff felt overworked while still underachieving the standard they had cherished for this new unit, but also that Green House was not able to function to its full capacity of 22 beds. The resulting concern led to such levels of discontent that management found themselves confronted in dispute with the staff unions. Although eventually staffing levels were ameliorated and a 'bank' set up to facilitate the use of staff across the new locality, the ill-feeling and mistrust took a long time to die away. In fact, it was not until the advent of yet another (able and team-minded) charge nurse that Green House renewed its positive vision of service. This, coincidentally, proved an appropriate moment for the introduction of the DCM tool (as part of the Springton DCM project,) which I had first used at Green House.

Finally, Green House was planned, designed, built and began to function during a period of momentous Health Service reforms. The mental health unit of the District Health Authority began the reprovision programme within the former ethos of top-down, rational, strategic planning, relatively generously resourced from top-sliced funding through 'capital programmes'. By the time it opened, the new internal market structures of the health service (the 'purchaser/provider split') were becoming a reality, and the unit was in 'shadow Trust status' – that is, the whole organisation was learning to function in different ways informed by a new and urgent appreciation of resource limitation. Just fourteen months after Green House opened, the new Springton Mental Health Care NHS Trust came into being on 1 April 1992. Therefore, from inception to functioning, the staff and managers involved with the Green House service had lived and worked through one of the most momentous periods of change in the Health Service since 1948, through it all striving to keep alive the initial vision of a facility to provide care 'in the community.'

Yet it would appear that not only did the community not want this particular manifestation of 'care', but they actually wanted something quite different: they wanted the old St John's hospital back – for 'geriatric' care. The Health Authority exercised enlightened despotism in forcing through (at considerable expense in a period of retrenchment) a new facility for clients with dementia, and achieved a good part of what they had set out to do. Therefore not only were the clients' voices (the service users) absent from the planning and provision process because their views were never solicited, but the wishes of the very 'community' for whom this care was being provided was actively disregarded as, justified by faith in their own greater wisdom, the

Health Authority heroically won the battle of the municipal potting shed.

Idealism in strategic planning and persistence in following through despite the odds are much to be admired. But both are better supported by being rooted in the concerns and preoccupations of those most affected. For these tend not to go away. Over time they emerge in new forms and require to be addressed. People do not stop having a point of view just because it has been disregarded – or, indeed, never been regarded as existing at all! So, having set the scene at Green House, let us now turn our attention to the hitherto ignored perspective of the clients themselves.

# CHAPTER 4

# What the clients said

*Interviewing elderly people with dementia in a day-hospital and an in-patient unit produced four overall themes: their awareness of themselves and their situation; the importance for good or ill of other people; the losses which preoccupied them; and their experience of dependence.*

It is time now to look at the actual concerns and preoccupations of the people for whom Green House had ostensibly been set up: the clients of the service. The themes that emerged from a content analysis of their interview transcripts fell into four main categories: their awareness, the significance of other people, a variety of issues around loss, and their experience of dependence. I shall examine each of these in turn, as far as possible through the words of the clients themselves. And I shall look at some of the memory-stories to see how we can extrapolate meaning through seeking the metaphorical content in such stories. For it is not sufficient simply to say that long-term memory is relatively better preserved, and that therefore this is why clients tell stories of their earlier life. The question we have to answer is, why this particular story at this particular time? We need to ask what it could be telling us about, and why it might be useful to understand this.

I have made use of extensive quotation from the interview transcripts. I want, as it were, to step back and let the clients speak for themselves. Some of the clients to whom I make several references I have given names, but not their own names. Since these were not monologues, the words of both interviewer and respondent feature in these quotations. I have simply labelled the interviewer 'I', and the respondent 'R'. I have tried to present the clients' voiced concerns with a gentle hand, in order to leave intact their 'surplus of meaning' for the reader to savour first-hand (Ricoeur 1976). This was particularly important in regard to the first theme, awareness. For to listen to the client respondents' explicit recognition of their situation and their problems is an exercise in awareness for the hearer also.

## Awareness

### Awareness of interview

I should begin by saying that of the 22 clients I interviewed from both the day-hospital and the in-patient unit at Green House, nine (almost half) demonstrated their understanding of the interview situation by referring to it directly during the course of the interview. They were cognizant of the nature of the situation: that their views were being canvassed:

> I.   It's really nice that you've agreed to do this because it's going to be very helpful to me.
>
> R.   Yes. What is it you want to know?

Another person said:

> You're very welcome to ask me at any time for what I know might be very helpful. If there's anything you want to learn about from me, you're welcome.
>
> Very glad to be of help.

One day-hospital client stated at the outset of the interview:

> I understand quite a lot really.

He then added the caveat:

> So I would appreciate the fullest confidence.

A client who was held as an in-patient under a section of the Mental Health Act said at the end of the interview:

R.  Just to show that I do know a little bit about it, but I have found quite a lot of things that I thought I'd forgot about.

I.  Well thank you very much for doing that, that was really helpful.

R.  All the very best, my dear, and good luck to you.

At the end of each interview I fed back to each client my understanding of what they had said – using their own words as far as I could remember them – in just the same way that I read my notes back to all my other respondents. Their reaction was invariably gracious. It seemed to have been a genuinely pleasurable experience for many of them:

I.  …having a little chat here, just the two of us.

R.  Enjoying it, aren't we? … I think that's about the lot. Shall we go for a little walk now?

One client sought reassurance that her contribution would be useful to me:

I.  Very interesting talk, Janet. I'm very grateful.

R.  Well, you're quite welcome.

I.  It will be very useful to me.

R.  Will it?

I.  Yes, it will.

R.  That's all right then.

She also showed a real understanding of my wanting to capture a diversity of perspectives on Green House:

I.  People are very helpful and they share with me how they see things and I add them all up – how everybody sees things – and it gets very interesting.

R.  It does, I suppose. They can't all think alike.

A feature of several interviews was the way clients reacted to the opening rituals: the asking of permission to interview, the reassurance about confidentiality, the reading and signing of the consent form, and the attaching of the small microphone to their lapel. These formed a prelude which was evidently seen as a boost to (perhaps flagging) self-esteem. 'Samuel' in the day-hospital, already with a confirmed reputation as a raconteur, accepted the interview invitation with a considerable show of graciousness. He would be only too glad to be of help. He also signed the consent form for his interview himself (for some clients their carer or key worker signed for them) and this with no little panache – putting his spectacles on the end of his nose, reading the form, and filling in the date (correctly) under his signature without even having to ask what it was. Several clients did this, and it seemed as if the 'normal person' status conferred by being asked for an interview unlocked the doors of short-term memory temporarily. It was significant that none of them made reference to the 'reality orientation' board on the wall for the date; indeed, the interviews were usually carried out around the corner, where they could not have seen it anyway.

A second noticeable feature of these interviews with clients was their reaction to 'noises off'. Minimising confusing stimuli for those who suffer from dementia has for some time been recognised as contributing positively to clients' sense of well-being, and to their ability to orient themselves in the environment (Netten 1993). I, too, noticed during these interviews that where noise or commotion intervened, sometimes a client's perhaps previously reasonably coherent train of thought often degenerated into fragmentary and confused phrases with little seeming association.

For instance, 'Mary' was a day-hospital client who was already distressed as she did her best to explain how she hated the slippers she had been given to wear, and wanted her shoes back, because she was afraid that she would have to stay in Green House permanently. The substitution of slippers for shoes she interpreted symbolically. And she was obviously afraid of some of the other clients who were wandering around. She said tearfully that she did not want to come to

Green House, that she wanted to go back to her 'real home' (she was in residential care). It was noticeable that when a wandering client approached, her confusion increased.

However, those clients who seemed happier or were observably more assertive in their behaviour dealt with interruptions with equanimity, and even included discussion of them in the conversation. One redoubtable woman in the in-patient facility dismissed a rather tactlessly shouted invitation by one of the care staff to come and join in a game of softball – they could see we were talking together quietly in our corner:

R. Playing that stupid game!

I. They're playing softball: stupid game?

R. Yes. I'm not gonna look at 'em. [Raising her voice in reply to them:] No – there's not room for us and we ain't coming down there!

Another interview in the day-hospital was interrupted by a wandering client who was often quite physically aggressive. The client I was interviewing had a painful arm as the result of a fall at home, and was obviously a little nervous of being approached on her 'poorly' side. Nevertheless, fortified by the cigarette she had taken the opportunity of smoking 'round the corner', she was able to converse happily on the likely objective of the wanderer and whether or not she might be going to the toilet. Her speech remained as coherent as before.

So all these interviewees clearly demonstrated their awareness of the present moment – both the interview situation, and their surroundings. We should not find this surprising. After all, if people with dementia were as oblivious to everything as is commonly believed, why would noise and commotion, the aggressive stance of another person, or a tactless intervention bring forth these reactions? To be disturbed by events in the environment one must be aware of them.

*Awareness of own confusion*

A third of the clients also showed they were aware of their own cognitive problems: their sense of confusion and forgetfulness. They spoke of it in different ways, some excusatory and some apologetic. Two clients in the in-patient facility put it this way:

> Would like to have had a chat with you properly, but you see I wouldn't know what to talk about, not what they're interested in … If there was, there's something I couldn't say – I haven't the foggiest notion, because I haven't got any notions.

> My trouble really is myself … My problem is myself, have to remember … I forget, you see … I'm not much of a one to talk, because I don't know.

Another client receiving 'respite care' referred to herself as having 'double mixtures'. When I asked if she could say a bit more about this, she replied:

> Yes. I do get fed up with it. Mmm.

Regular clients of the day-hospital were similarly candid:

> Well, I should say that I was not an authority to handle information because if I was I should be happy to … If I was an authority I should feel I was in a position to deal with it and anything else. I should feel that it would be helpful to you to know – I should do that.

One referred to what happened every time the minibus called to bring him to Green House:

> as soon as they arrive [laughing] – I call it 'the waggon!' – they come for me and they come to the door as though they've known me for years. 'Are you ready?' – and they are so patient with me and they come in to see if I've left everything all right. I understand that – they're so conscientious. They see if the fire's out or if I've turned the gas off, and all that sort of thing, which I appreciate because

I haven't got a great memory now – you don't when you get older.

Another also excused her memory's inadequacies as being the result of age:

You know, you do get sort of vague when you'm getting older, and don't know where everything's to, you know.

Not surprisingly, given this awareness of their own confusion, six clients showed evidence of low self-esteem in their interviews, using self-deprecatory remarks and apologising for their confused state. For example, 'Rose' who 'had no notions' continued by saying:

I can't – I'm a terrible person.

When describing a 'chat' with a member of staff, she could not remember a place name:

Terribly rude of me, I dare say ... I can't remember any place names, isn't it terrible?

She ended the interview by saying:

Well, I wish I could have made myself – I could have – been more interesting.

James whose 'problem was himself' went on to say:

I'm not much of a one to talk because I don't know.

Another in-patient who was able to speak often only in partial sentences, and whose phrases would end in sudden long silences during which she appeared to lose her train of thought, said:

I'm not being very helpful!

Janet was a day-hospital client who wept over the loss of her husband, and the fact that her children now lived far away. Her interview was full of remarks such as: 'I can't change it', 'What else could I do?', 'I just accept it'.

Another woman in the day-hospital, whose speech was prolific but who became confused with her own confusion, echoed this theme:

Oh, what am I talking about – the, err, oh, I can't say it now – how stupid – oh, I can't repeat it … I'm so stupid I can't repeat it.

### Awareness of own approaching death

Several of the clients I interviewed referred to their own approaching death. In particular three of the clients who had been brought into the in-patient facility for respite care spoke of this. It was as if being brought in to stay (as opposed to attending the day-hospital) emphasised 'the beginning of the end' in their minds. Jane was a respite client who recounted her husband's final illness several times, saying how much he had suffered and how glad she had been for him to be released from his pain:

R.   And he's waiting for me in heaven.

I.   I'm sure he is.

R.   That was his last talk.

I.   He told you and you remember that.

R.   I'm looking forward to him coming back –

I.   Being together again –

R.   That's right … When I get to heaven I shall thank God very much.

The serenity on her face as she said this indicated a genuine pleasure at the thought of being reunited with her husband. But also by analogy she was expressing the relief that death brings from present suffering. She had been glad for her husband when he had been released from pain; the inference appeared to be that she would also appreciate being released from her own condition. Jane was physically not very well, as she suffered from a variety of conditions in addition to her confusion. Life was not easy for her, therefore, and death had more than one thing to commend it.

For another client this preoccupation was a recurrent feature of his periods as an in-patient. He told me that he was aware of his wife's need for a rest, because she had a job as well as having to look after him. So he came into Green House for her sake – so that she should have a break. However, he said that he never wanted to come in, even though the staff were very pleasant to him, and took him out for walks, which he liked. It was noticeable that this client did not mix in any way with the other in-patients, preferring to stay in his room, or to stay beside the staffroom, talking to the staff. He said that he had problems sleeping at Green House, because he always had the same nightmare every time he came in. He dreamt that he was being shut up in a box from which he could not get out. He spoke so sadly, as he told of the terrible sweating panic that this dream engendered. This was what made him afraid to go to sleep while an in-patient. The fact that he evidently found the presence of the other clients (who were very much more disabled than he was) so disturbing, and clung to the much younger and 'normal' staff, together with his love of being taken out walking, all integrated with this recurrent nightmare. As he spoke it seemed clear that the box might be a coffin. When I discussed this with Tom Kitwood later, he also immediately inter-preted the dream in this way – as a fear of approaching death.

For yet another respite client it seemed that her sense of not having long to live was linked with her awareness of her own condition. This was the patient who described her confusion as having 'double mixtures':

R.   I do get fed up with it.

I.   You get fed up?

R.   Mmm. It won't be much longer, 'cos I'm getting on old now.

*Age as a bid for recognition and understanding*

Age was used by several of the clients to explain or excuse their for-getfulness or confusion. But age had a dual valency. That is, beyond a certain stage the 'decrepitude' flavour of old age could become 'venerability', carrying with it a sense of having lasted the course – achieved a marathon. It was therefore also a reason for pride and a way of bolstering flagging self-esteem, which was a feature of many of the interviews. So in these clients' interviews the concept of age could be used like a pivot chord in music: belonging to two keys and facilitating the smooth modulation from one to the next – from minor (forgetfulness, confusion) to major (a statement of identity and achievement). For example, Samuel in the day-hospital, after confiding that he knew he was getting forgetful, used it in precisely this way:

R.   I'm 80 odd, you know – born in 1903.

I.   80 –?

R.   I was born in 1903!

I.   Gosh!

R.   Didn't you know that?

I.   No, I didn't know that. 1903 – that's a long time ago.

It was interesting to note that all the clients, when referring to their age, defined it by the year of their birth. The process of autobiographical life-review would appear to require a definite beginning, and in each case it led the client into the telling of their own life-story – the narrative of their identity. In this way the stating of the year seemed to serve the function of 'once upon a time'. Samuel continued by talking of the place of his birth, now no longer in existence, together with the sort of small local details and anecdotes which could only be known to someone who had been there at that time. Since I was less than half his age, it seemed almost as if he was laying claim to some status as the holder of privileged and esoteric knowledge.

Another day-hospital respondent referred to her great age with poetic licence:

R.   I'm over a hundred.

I.   Over a hundred?

R.   Well, 91. Yes, so I'm getting on … I say can't do anything out for my – I'm old enough for anything – old 900!

Yet another, who was confined to a wheelchair after a stroke, said that he would value what he called 'an old-fashioned approach' at Green House. 'I'm an old man' he said by way of explanation. His physical dependency and communication difficulties were evidently depressing him, and his eyes would fill with tears. It seemed that this was an indirect request for a gentler pace of interaction, having regard for his age and infirmity.

## Identity as a bid for individual recognition

As we get older we all tend to review and reconstruct our memories of our past life in order to try to make sense of it, and to understand (or remind ourselves) who we are.

> The most important aspect of autobiographical memory in old age is represented by the processes of life review. The function of autobiographical memory in maintaining the self and in leading to further developments of self – the emergence of integrity – is of critical importance for at least some people. It seems likely that the purpose of life review and the role of autobiographical memory in this process are determined more by the existential problems set by the past and the nature of current circumstances than by any predetermined cognitive process (Conway 1990).

For the Green House clients, the memories of the past which were prompted by the nature of current circumstances were selected, and perhaps reconstructed, in a life review process whose aim would appear to be to forge a strong, 'worthwhile', valuable historical identity as a bulwark against the fear of helplessness, confusion, dependence, and its concomitant stigma. For example, in her interview one of the day-hospital clients included stories which accounted for her maiden name and both her married names. In other words, three distinct identity markers were given great prominence.

And there were other topics relating to the question of identity, or personhood, spontaneously generated in these interviews. In particular, seven of the respondents (both men and women) spoke at some length about their working life. Samuel emphasised the fact that he was a 'craftsman' (a maker of musical instruments) as against 'mere labouring' – because this was a more 'worthwhile' job. The stories he told about both his strict father and his demanding but paternalistic boss painted a clear picture of the uncompromising patriarchy in which he had grown up. He was saying something fundamental about his sense of identity by explaining the demanding nature of his value-system, and how he had acquired it. He was a man with high expectations of himself, particularly with regard to being responsible for his own work and decisions, and it was now hard for him not to be able to live up to them as he believed he should. He was therefore explaining why it was hard for him to be dependent on the kindness of others, and why he saw it as inherently stigmatising.

He then continued to tell the story of an old and deaf craftsman whom, as a young apprentice, he had joined in baiting and teasing:

> We had a fella – old, had a beard, – we used to call him 'fairy' … We were real lads in those days. 'Fairy!' And he was deaf, very deaf. After [the boss] brought people round, we used to go to 'Fairy' and tell him what they were talking about – and it was all made up! Poor old 'Fairy'! In the end he'd get – a lad, get a piece of wood, and he'd hit you; you'd have to get out of his way. Very, very old craftsman, but deaf, gone deaf … They used to call it mischievous, but – 'Fairy Lore' – his name was Fred Law, and we called him 'Fairy Lore' [laughter].

Samuel knew how people treat those who are handicapped, and how they could take advantage of them. Fred Law had been reliant on others to tell him what had been said, because he was deaf. The visitors to the company had, in fact, been shown the craftsmen and their work with pride by the managing director. But the 'lads' had obviously told Fred a different story. Significantly he must have realised what they were doing, because he became angry and tried to hit them. Samuel remembered how he himself participated in the baiting of a deaf old man, whom he always referred to as a 'craftsman' (like himself) – thereby according him the status of his expertise and experience. The story tells us that these did not save him from the teasing of the younger ones. It was his deafness they saw, not his experience. And they called him what, despite being ostensibly a play on words, was in fact rather a derogatory name (even granted that 'fairy' then probably did not have its contemporary connotations).

Samuel would seem to be explaining why it was so important to him to relate his achievements and to construct (or reconstruct) his identity through autobiographical memories: he was not merely an elderly man with dementia (the reason for his attendance at Green House). Like 'Fairy Lore' he was a venerable craftsman too, and his experience and knowledge were of an older vintage than his present frailty. He laughed quite a lot while telling this story, but at the end his voice seemed to express some doubt as to whether 'mischievous' was really the right word to describe his actions. Jokes can be a safer and more acceptable way of dealing with feelings and memories that come too close for comfort.

Samuel juxtaposed this story with another about asking his boss for a 'raise'. Money is both a measure and a symbol of value or worth. He was talking about it directly after remembering how he and his fellows had 'belittled' the old deaf craftsman until he had resorted to picking up a piece of wood and trying to hit his tormentors as a way of asserting that he was not of so little value that he could be mocked with impunity. Samuel seemed to be referring to the powerlessness engendered by not being able to stand up for oneself by virtue of disability or frailty. His story of how he asked his boss for a rise was therefore highlighting the fact that those who had power would not acknowledge worth unless it was in their interest to do so:

> And I remember going in for a raise in wages – cheeky – the boss nearly fell down when I asked him – 'What do you want? What do you want?' – trying to belittle you.

By analogy, if you were a 'client' with 'dementia', your worth would be acknowledged only in those terms. This could be the fear that lay behind such attempts to present an individual and valuable identity. It was the only 'bargaining power' that Samuel and those in his position now possessed.

James would consistently show the medal he had been given as headboy of his school (famous locally), and the silver whistle attached to it, which his children had used to gnaw on when cutting their teeth. The little teeth-marks were still visible. He was claiming the identities of his youth: exemplary pupil and 'achiever', and father of a family.

The subject of grandchildren was another identity and status-reinforcing topic which occurred in several interviews. 'Vera' spoke about her meals in the day-hospital:

> ...the sweet as well. My little grandson keeps asking 'What have you had for afters?' He calls it 'afters!' The sweet comes – so I told him. 'Oh, you are lucky!' he keeps saying – because he likes sweets – the little monkey!

The discussion of such a mundane and practical subject as 'afters' immediately brought her grandson to mind, and, despite digressions, it was to this subject that she returned:

> R. And I tell them [the other clients] about my grandson [laughter] – the little monkey he is!
>
> I. You are very fond of him, I think.
>
> R. Oh, yes. And I miss my grandsons which are in Bradford. I have another two there.
>
> I. Bradford. Bradford-in-the-Vale?
>
> R. No. Bradford in Yorkshire. Yes, they are living there, and I miss them.

Michael in the in-patient unit explained frankly that he would rather be at home than at Green House:

> ...because I have six grandchildren.

But the most cogent expression of the importance of the whole question of identity was by Norma, who now resided permanently in the in-patient facility. Her speech was not only impeded by breath-lessness, but also by the fact that she was unable ever to finish a sentence. She would begin, and progress as far as the key word which was needed to make sense of what had gone before – and then she would be unable to find it. She and I persevered together through several such 'cliff-hangers', to the point where she said that she had been in Green House 'a very, very, very long...' As I supplied 'a long time?' she began to gesticulate in the direction of the other residents.

She was already becoming tired and more breathless, and I was considering bringing the interview to a close, when she made an enormous effort, sat up straight, and said one of her few complete sentences:

I need to be me!

This was said with great vehemence, and she beat her chest with her right fist as she said 'me!' After this she collapsed back, exhausted, on the sofa where she and I were sitting together. I double-checked with her what she had just said:

I.  To be you?

R.  Yes.

I.  Do you feel – is that difficult: to be you, to be yourself?

R.  Yes ... So much talking and that, and I just say to you – and that's all you can have.

She had expended all her energy on getting this one, crucial statement across, and could do no more. In the context of the large and 'barn-like' (as more than one person described it) in-patient sitting-room, with the other residents either wandering around or sitting in apathy, and with some of them calling out, her meaning was extraordinarily clear. How to hang on to a sense of self and individuality, when all about and all within seemed to be disintegrating? Perhaps she had voiced the prime issue for all of the clients: 'I need to be me!' In searching for a title for this book, I found her words seemed the most appropriate.

## Changing awareness

The 22 clients I interviewed could be divided into three groups: those who attended the day-hospital, those who were in the in-patient facility, and those who used both the day-hospital and the in-patient facility for respite care. Eleven were day-hospital clients, six were in-patients, and five had experience of both day-hospital and in-patient facilities. This was, therefore, a very small sample from which to generalise about changes in client awareness relating to whether they were in receipt of day-care or part-time or full-time in-patient care. Nevertheless, even from this small group of clients a certain picture seemed to emerge from an examination of the issues and topics uppermost in their minds at interview when asked about their experience of Green House. For there was some variation in the topics raised by each group.

The day-hospital clients raised more issues. Partly this was because there were more of them. But partly, perhaps, also it resulted from a broader experience of present environment and, no doubt, from a generally lesser handicap in communication. The topics covered by this group were as follows: communication; familiarity; looking forward to coming to the day-hospital; identity and related topics including working life, family and grandchildren; people, social contact and friendship; refuge and support; bereavement and loss; age; dependence; dignity; resignation; isolation; anxiety about the future; low self-esteem; appreciation of physical care; own physical pains and problems; fear and absence of trust; home; needing to be needed; a sense of desertion.

The topics found in the interviews with those in the in-patient facility were fewer, and seemed to correspond to their altered status, as having finally lost their place in the outside community. They were: awareness of own approaching death; loss; awareness of others in control; home; boredom; the parental model and strictness (the word as well as the concept); awareness of, and apologies for, their own communication problems; low self-esteem; people (staff and residents); family; gender; isolation; escape.

Those clients who had experience of both the day-hospital and the in-patient facilities (the respite care clients) provided a variation – with significant additions – to those covered by the clients in the in-patient facility. They were in a certain sense at the half-way point between the first two groups. Being admitted as an in-patient to Green House for respite care, or under Mental Health Act section, could be interpreted as marking a milestone in the process of dementia for any given individual client. They had not yet had to accept the final loss of independence – hence the topic of privacy and peace, and the awareness of being detained under section. The full list of topics was as follows: loss; awareness of own confusion; bereavement; awareness of communication problems; low self-esteem; awareness of being sectioned under the Mental Health Act; awareness of own approaching death; home; family; privacy and peace; boredom; loneliness; a sense of isolation; anger/violence/aggression.

## The importance of other people

As clients had demonstrated their awareness of themselves, their confusion and their situation, it was not surprising that they also spoke a great deal of their awareness of other people and the importance of congenial company. In fact, the subject of social contact featured in half the interviews, and in all these interviews people and friendship were also the first subjects to be mentioned:

I. Life here at Green House when you come here, how does that feel to you?

R. Very pleasant ... Yes, the people are very nice.

I. You like the people?

R. Yes, I do.

A minute later in the same interview:

I. What about the various things that you do here at Green House? Which of those is particularly enjoyable for you?

R. Well, I think – rather hard to explain – but being among people, talking to them.

Clients discussed the importance of other people in various ways. A third of them spoke directly of how people need each other, and of how it is people who make life worthwhile. For instance, Samuel said:

R. I look forward to coming. And I've met charming people here, just like coming home again ... I like the people. I like the place, but I like the people – attractive people, nice people.

I. It's the people that's important?

R.  It is very important anywhere really.

I.  That's true.

R.  People that make life worth living.

Another day-hospital client who had been very disabled by a stroke, so that his speech as well as his mobility were affected, replied to the question 'Which things do you enjoy here?':

R.  I've good friends here.

I.  Good friends.

R.  Good friends ... It's a very good family.

I.  Like a family?

R.  To feel confidence and to have confidence.

I.  So it gives you confidence to feel among friends?

R.  Yes.

The importance of friendship and familiarity was echoed by Vera:

R.  Oh, I like to come here ... I like all the people around me because they are known to me.

I.  You have got to know them?

R.  Oh yes, they are all friendly, very friendly ...

I.  Sounds as if you look forward to coming.

R.  Oh yes, to see all the old faces, yes. They are all kind ... I just like the people. I like everybody here – they are so familiar to me.

Two day-hospital clients went on to explain why people were so important, in terms of the necessity of interdependence: 'We all rely on one another, you know.' This was a significant issue arising from the client interviews, to which we will return.

'Edna' who attended both the day-hospital and the in-patient facility for respite care, said of coming to Green House:

I think it gives me an opportunity to mix with other
members of the fraternities, which otherwise I shouldn't ... I

think it is very important that we should mix with one another and learn to appreciate what other people do for us and give up – especially when they give up – err – spare time.

(This was a reference to the staff, whom she was able to describe as 'the people who come and give their services here'.) Edna spoke very slowly and had considerable difficulty finding words; she left extremely long pauses between phrases and even words, and this could mean that she would lose the thread of what she had been trying to say. On other occasions, however, she was obviously carefully reformulating it, and here she produced this summary:

I do appreciate the fact that this gives me an opportunity of meeting many people who otherwise I wouldn't meet.

Interestingly, her care scores in the DCM observations were higher when she was in the in-patient facility than when she was in the day-hospital: 'fair' in the day-hospital, rising to 'good' when an in-patient on respite care. This differentiated her from the other three clients interviewed, who experienced both day-hospital and in-patient care at Green House. Perhaps this was related to her reply when asked if there was anything she did not like at Green House:

No, I don't think so. Err – I always look at it from this point of view: if there's something that I don't like, no doubt there are other people who don't like me! And it might enable me to broaden my own horizons.

This was a remarkably courageous and positive attitude to her situation. In fact, her social background as a retired professional woman was different to that of almost all the other clients at that time, and she was seeking a positive handle to enable her to accept the differences. Her quietness and slowness of speech meant that often in the jollity of the day-hospital she appeared rather left to the side of things. In the slower atmosphere of the in-patient facility she perhaps found opportunities for relating to other people (especially the staff) in the more reflective fashion which suited her.

Roy, a day-hospital client, spoke of friendship as the most important thing for him in coming to Green House:

I.  Which things do you enjoy here?

R.  Oh yes, I've good friends here.

I.  Good friends?

R.  Good friends … Friendship I enjoy. Hope I'll go on enjoying.

I.  Right.

R.  They treat me with …

I.  They treat you well?

R.  They speak to me.

So in Roy's interview there was an explicit recognition of a crucial characteristic of friendship:

They speak to me.

This was particularly poignant, given that, as we shall see later, the ability to communicate verbally was used by staff as a measure of clients' awareness. Being spoken to is seen here by the client as the indicator of friendship. Given the importance of social contact for clients, together with their awareness of their own confusion, it was understandable that communication should have been such a significant topic in these interviews. More than a quarter of the clients I interviewed referred to it directly; for instance Samuel:

After being living with my daughter, and I – it's only one of us now, my wife died, her mother died – and she goes out to work and I am on my own. It's a great pleasure to come here and meet people who are sensible enough to talk – you know what I mean.

This could be interpreted either as referring to the staff, or perhaps to the other clients, with whom the respondent could be seen as sharing not only an analogous present predicament but also a generational common experience. These were people who had lived through the same historical public events, experienced many of the same life events, and who had also travelled through the great changes and developments of the twentieth century. The potentially problematic nature of communication for people with dementia underlines the need for any commonality of experience that can facilitate it. Samuel exercised his gifts as a raconteur in an ongoing process of life-review: he had led an interesting life and acquired some unusual skills, and he delighted in sharing these stories with whomever would listen. His care scores in the DCM observations were consistently high, averaging 'very good', and in all instances the behaviour which chiefly characterised his time at Green House was social interaction. Because good verbal communication was still open to him, and was also rewarding for his audience, he received affirming and validating reinforcement for the strong historical identity which he wove from his autobiographical stories.

A woman who attended the day-hospital from a residential home, and who therefore was not deprived of company in her 'home' situation, nevertheless gave priority to the importance of communication in her enjoyment of coming to Green House:

I.   What about the various things that you do here at Green House. Which of those is particularly enjoyable to you?

R.   Well, I think – rather hard to explain – but being among people – talking to them ... yes, talking to people.

Vera echoed this:

I.   Anything that you particularly like when you come here?

R.   Just the people.

I.   The people.

R.   Yes, and when we talk.

I.   So you talk here quite a lot?

R.   Oh yes, when I met the people whom I know, we talk then.

But for some, communication was a negative experience:

I.   What about the people here, do you feel happy with them here?

R. Well, I don't know these people here.

I. You don't know them.

R. No, no. No. I'm quite happy to have a word with them if I choose to, but no, I don't have anything to do with them really.

I. You don't.

R. No, no.

I. Because you don't know them?

R. Well, err, not being acquainted with them for quite a long time...

Out of the importance of communication, then, came also the critical issue of familiarity. To know and be known was the prerequisite for meaningful and valuable communication; and communication was the prime means whereby identity could be preserved. Familiarity – of people, places, and things – was also in itself a crucial support for a sense of identity and of control over one's life. Familiar surroundings and people reinforce autobiographical memory, encourage independence, and facilitate meaningful communication. For Vera familiarity was the first reason she gave for liking Green House:

R. Oh, I like to come here.

I. You like it?

R. Yes. I like all the people around me because they are known to me.

I. You have got to know them?

R. Oh yes. They are all friendly, very friendly. I kept saying at home 'Is it Green House?' [Laughing]

I. Sounds as if you look forward to coming.

R. Oh yes. To see all the old faces, yes.

She continued in the same vein:

I. What are the days like for you here?

R.  Oh, I just like – I like the people. I like everybody here – they are so familiar to me.

I.  And that's important: familiarity?

R.  Oh yes, yes.

I.  So when you're here and you are talking to people – the people that you are familiar with – how does that make you feel?

R.  Oh, just as my family – yes, just like a family.

Interestingly, familiarity was not a topic that came up in the interviews with those in the in-patient facility. For those day-hospital clients who found Green House a positive experience, the reassurance of regular social contact with the same familiar people and setting was perhaps facilitated by being able to hang on to other familiar aspects of their lives. This would appear to support the Green House service's commitment to keeping clients 'in the community' for as long as possible.

## Potential feelings of loneliness and isolation

As most of the day-hospital clients had relatively greater verbal communication skills, it seemed clear from what they said that Green House day-hospital answered an important area of concern in providing a warm and welcoming social environment, which observably facilitated much positive social interaction. But by implication the lack of meaningful contact with other people could be loneliness and a sense of isolation. Some of those I spoke to made this connection explicit, some did not. It was, however, a common topic across each of the three groups of client respondents: day-hospital clients, in-patient clients, and day-hospital clients who also experienced in-patient 'respite' care. Several people explicitly acknowledged this overriding importance for them of being with other people – the rescue from loneliness. It was described on a warm, sunny afternoon by one woman attending the day-hospital like this:

I'm glad they brought me here because, well, really – cold wind – I'm glad somebody sort of found me. I didn't really

> know which way I had to go, you know – but when you're
> on your own it's – I don't know.

The 'cold wind' referred to here would seem to be a metaphor for the chill of isolation and confusion, as opposed to the warmth of human contact.

Sarah (a widow) was even more explicit about the day-hospital:

> I like it, to tell you the truth. I'm on me own all day long, my husband's at work all day, I've got no – well, I've got one married daughter and she lives away from home – so I'm a bit lonely; so I'd much rather come up here than sit indoors moping all day long.

But the significance of social contact and the manner of its acceptability could be highly individually variable. Janet in the day-hospital expressed clearly what was implicit in the interviews of several of the clients, that is, a sense of being the 'odd one out' – of not belonging. This was expressed in the context of not fitting in with the other clients, and the reason given was the lack of a shared background:

I.   You said that you find it dull in here at times.

R.   Well, I do at times because I haven't got much in common ... A lot of people don't know much about farming now, see. And they don't take any interest in it. When I'm going out places I look over hedges and see what there is about – see what animals there are about and all that sort of thing – which other people don't do. It's not their line of business.

A little later she added:

> I don't belong to any Women's Institute or anything of that, you see ... And I don't know if I want to. I don't belong to Mothers' Union or anything like that. I've never had time for that.

Given that day-hospital outings were relatively rare and did not in any case include visiting farms, Janet seemed to be expressing symbolically her feeling of not belonging in the group. The Women's Institute and the Mothers' Union could be seen as analogies of the 'club' atmosphere of the day-hospital. Janet had her own individual identity which she was trying to hang on to. Never having been a 'joiner,' she now felt it inappropriate to be in a situation where she was seemingly expected to be part of a group, with which she felt no common interest. She might also have been recognising the nature of the day-hospital and therefore rejecting its appropriateness for her.

Similarly, when talking about Green House, Edna, attending the in-patient unit for 'respite' care, suddenly recounted how she had been the only girl in a family of boys when she was little, and that she had not liked that. Given the juxtaposition of ideas, and the fact that most of her fellow in-patients were evidently considerably more handicapped than she was, it was conceivable that this was also a reference to a feeling of being 'the odd one out'.

But even in the more congenial and stimulating atmosphere of the day-hospital, for some clients interpersonal contacts could be very negative. For example, Mary, a day-hospital client, was clearly perennially uneasy in a group environment, preferring to stay away from group activities and smiling only occasionally when in one-to-one conversations with staff. Her isolation from the group was self-imposed, therefore, although she clearly valued the gentle personal attention she received from staff. She was obviously extremely wary of those clients who wandered or called out. Throughout the interview she was constantly looking around nervously as people moved towards or around her, or called out from a different part of the lounge. She was particularly frightened of one other woman client, Daisy, who could not speak and who wandered incessantly. Daisy was also often aggressive, and would wander near to someone and then strike them – hard. Mary's fear was therefore well founded. And she had reached the point of constantly looking toward the glass door between the in-patient dining-room and the day-hospital lounge, as it was from the in-patient area that Daisy attended the day-hospital, while in for respite care to give her husband a break. Mary's short-term memory loss did not protect her from remembering previous attacks and therefore dreading another.

She spoke constantly about how she did not like coming to Green House and how she wished to be taken back to her 'real home'.

Here the sense of isolation was heightened by actual fear. The respondent's continual and tearful reference to her home could be seen as a desire for refuge:

R. I got to be taken home.

I. You've got to be taken home?

R. Home. Not – my right home.

I. Not your real home.

R. No.

I. Do you look forward to being taken away then?

R. Yeh. Won't take you home. No, no. Not my home. [Crying] … Shall have to stay here altogether … I don't want to stay … No. No.

Clients spoke a lot about their families. But for some the question of family relationships sometimes had a darker meaning. Pat spoke of how she no longer saw very much of her children:

> I've never seen much of the family, not since then. They used to come down on a Sunday evening and come in for a while, and then they didn't seem quite so eager to come so they haven't seen Mum [herself] for quite a while now … They got a bit fed up, I suppose, with coming our way – so they didn't come.

She seemed to be expressing a sense of desertion. It was in this way that the sense of isolation (which the DCM observations showed to be such a feature of the in-patient facility) was reinforced, as clients' confusion and communication problems (which already isolated them from other people) could sometimes make it increasingly less rewarding for their nearest and dearest to spend time with them. For someone who had, by her own admission, spent all her life looking after and working for her family, such isolation left her bereft of a meaning to her life, and having retold the story of how 'they didn't seem quite so eager to come' she moved on to reiterate over and over again her anxiety to find something useful to do to help. It sounded as if she would have liked the Green House staff to provide her with a job, so that she could service their needs, and in this way fulfil her own. The significance of family relationships, therefore, also appeared to be about the need to be needed.

While this attitude of mind would seem possibly particularly true of women clients of that generation, in fact several of the male clients interviewed also chose to speak of their families, their children and grandchildren, both as defining their identity and with pride in achievement:

> Before they built the dental hospital I lived there, and I used to watch the students larking about when I was a little kid, never thinking that my own daughter would become a student there ... Jane has got a degree from there, you know!

The way so many of the client respondents likened their social contact at Green House to being 'like a family' could be seen in one way as an accolade. But from another point of view it could be interpreted as the expression of just such a need: that is, the longing for the irreplaceable close bonds of blood and affection, of which social mobility and infirmity had combined to rob them.

How far were these needs met for those who had definitively had to give up hearth and home, and were now in receipt of 'continuing care'? Michael, in the in-patient unit, was quite definite about why he was not happy at Green House. In fact this client had 'escaped' from there several times and been found wandering in the town. During the interview he asked if I had a car: 'I'm wondering how I could use you to drive me home.' I asked how he liked being at Green House:

R.  I don't particularly.

I.  You don't.

R.  Not particularly.

Later I checked this opinion out with him again:

I.  Is there anything that you like about being here?

R.  No.

I.   Nothing?

R.   I'd rather be at home.

I.   You'd rather be at home – right.

R.   Because I have six grandchildren.

On asking the staff about visits from his family it transpired that he did not receive any.

Rose, in the in-patient unit, phrased her sense of loneliness in terms of communication:

> I haven't had a lot of chat with people.

Rose's self-esteem seemed very low and she apologised continually for her confusion, of which she was very aware:

> If I could have got chatting to someone there – but you've obviously got to be interested in what you're talking about, haven't you? Leastways, that's how I think about it. That's the first thing – um – maybe one day I shall meet somebody interested – coming together … I don't know the first thing about this – nothing at all I could talk about because I couldn't tell.

Aware of her own confusion and communication difficulties, she was explaining why she 'hadn't had a lot of chat with people.' She was smiling and very happy throughout her interview, and clearly appreciated spending half-an-hour in one-to-one conversation. However, she seemed intent on excusing her self-evaluated incompetence by pointing out her lack of practice at Green House in 'chatting'.

Norma, who found it difficult to speak because of her breathlessness as much as her confusion, said that there were 'not a lot of people who will play with me.' Her very elderly husband had difficulty visiting Green House because he lived in an outlying village without transport. She had made friends with another woman in the in-patient facility (one of the survivors from the old psychiatric hospital) and they would sit side-by-side on the sofa after lunch, and doze together. Their communication was of necessity almost entirely non-verbal, consisting of smiles and occasionally putting an arm around each other.

As we shall see, the staff tended to evaluate clients' level of awareness in terms of their ability to communicate. In considering the importance of other people, clients were clearly very much aware of how their communication difficulties were the reason for their lack of social contact. Yet James voiced the inherent loneliness of the experience of dementia, irrespective of companionship; the 'unreachability' of being trapped in a world which no longer made sense:

> My problem is myself ... I got to go round here on my own, don't matter who is with me.

## Loss: a recurrent leitmotif in clients' discourse

Increasing age can be viewed as a succession of losses: loss of role, loss of spouse, of children, of friends, of faculties. With loss of memory and the confusion it entails comes also loss of identity and control, self-respect and independence. Perhaps it is not surprising, therefore, that loss in one form or another featured strongly in many of the client interviews. A quarter of the clients I interviewed spoke of bereavement, and several spoke of other losses.

In fact, this theme of loss occurred in all three groups of client interviews, although it seemed marginally more frequent among those in the in-patient facility. There were several different kinds of loss to which they referred. We have already seen that loss of faculties, in terms of confusion, forgetfulness, and communication difficulties, was a client concern, as were loss of a sense of identity and of self-esteem. Similarly we have heard about loss of family and a sense of desertion. Loss of independence and a sense of agency is some-thing we will be looking at in the next section. Here, then, I shall con-centrate on the loss of loved ones – bereavement – and the loss of home.

Before moving on to these areas of bereavement and 'home'. however, it is worth noting that several client respondents referred to loss obliquely by mentioning memories of other losses in their lives. Indeed, Winifred, who was interviewed when in the in-patient facility for respite care, recounted an old memory of having been burgled; that is, when asked about her experience at Green House one of the memories that came to the surface of her mind was of the trauma of having had what she possessed taken away from her:

R.  I know somebody went when I was just doing me – work. While I was doing that, they were there nicking. They stole the stuff and went on.

I.  They stole things? While you were working.

R.  Yes. While I were there doing it, they were doing theirs … Yes, somebody broke my doors and broke all – I never had nothing.

Winifred was already losing English, which had been her second language, and some of the words she sometimes used were in her native language. And she was aware of her own forgetfulness. She was the one who referred to her confusion as having 'double mixtures'. Being brought into Green House had taken away all her familiar life-cues, since she attended another day-hospital in Goughton, so that Green House was a totally unfamiliar environment to her.

James, who normally attended the day-hospital, had been admitted to Green House as an in-patient under a section of the Mental Health Act on the day of his interview. The seemingly para-doxical reason for this was that he had left his home and found his own way to Green House early that morning! This client was a sociable and conversational person and usually very much enjoyed his times at the day-hospital. It seemed more a tribute to his relationship with the staff and his own remaining orientation skills that he had voted with his feet and turned up early. However, it was somehow interpreted as evidence of confusion and of being 'at risk' through wandering the streets, and so he was 'sectioned.' The result was that he was ceaselessly wandering throughout the building in search of his hat, without which he would not have dreamt of going out. His hat seemed to represent not only his passport to getting out, but also somehow it was a part of himself. It was what he tipped and doffed in recognition to those around him. This was the client who said: 'My problem is myself.' He had been a travelling salesman:

> I can't get the right words and yet I've been tra – all my life
> I've been tra – ... travelling and talking and talking. Now I
> be here I can't tell you what that is – funny thing isn't it?
> That's the way I am.

Moreover, he was quite clear that something was now going on to keep him from travelling which was not being openly and honestly explained to him:

R.   Then, of course, can't travel.

I.   You can't?

R.   Well, that's what she told me. A lot of people can't travel
     now. You've got to get a licence and all sorts.

I.   A licence? Right.

R.   To travel. Can't go anywhere anymore. That's the way I see it
     anyway. I'm hanging about now ... and I've been here all
     this time – a dead loss. So that's the position, my dear, for
     me.

This loss of his freedom, together with the loss of his memory, seemed to be symbolised by his inability to find his hat:

> Now I've got this sort of thing. This is my own fault. That
> hat for instance. It's no value much, but it's my hat and I'm
> always putting it down and losing it. The thing I would like
> to do – all the things I've done here before – but, no – I
> can't go down to where I come from!

And again:

> I don't know where it is I want to go now, but I don't know
> which way to go. No, I don't.

In fact, this entire interview was was conducted 'on the hoof', as it were, since James indicated that he was most happy to be interviewed, but he could not sit down because he had to look for his hat. He seemed very glad of my company and enlisted my help in his quest. When this was brought to a successful conclusion in his room his face lit up with pleasure, and he seemed to have recovered more than his hat.

This symbolism of lost belongings or clothes recurred in another day-hospital client's interview. Mary was the client who wept to go to her 'real home', and kept looking with horror at her feet because her shoes had been replaced with comfortable slippers. The loss of her shoes she interpreted with foreboding as a deeply sinister move to keep her from going home. I shall look at the significance of the loss of home in a moment. Before that, however, I shall consider the most poignant experience of loss – that of bereavement.

### Bereavement

As we have seen, the presence of other people was probably the most significant feature of clients' experience of Green House – whether positive or negative. It was not surprising, therefore, that for several of them the loss of special people in their lives – bereavement – was also a major theme. Given the cognitive disruption of degenerative organic brain disorder, ancient bereavements were often expressed either as recent (as if they had just occurred) or in denial (as if the person was still alive), so that the anguish had to be revisited in all its freshness every time. Several clients wept as they spoke of dead husbands or parents. Yet they seemed also to be glad of the opportunity to speak of these feelings in the one-to-one intimacy of the interview situation. Although I was always vigilant of the need to conclude an interview if the person became distressed, on no occasion did I actually have to do this. Clients very clearly desired just such an opportunity to give expression to their grieving, and to be listened to.

In fact, bereavement was a major issue for a quarter of the clients interviewed – in particular three women, all of whom were widowed. Jane was interviewed while in for respite care:

> Stan [her late husband] won't be here every day … He's in the churchyard. He died from a cancer in his back passage –

and how he did suffer … Well, last year, I could see there
were something wrong with him. And then by the Friday he
was rushed off into Springton with cancer in his back
passage. And I went on my hands and knees – to thank God
for taking him because how he had suffered. You can
imagine that, can't you? … And he's waiting for me in
heaven.

Sarah spent almost the entire interview speaking of her dead father
and her dead husband. Indeed, there was some confusion at certain
points as to which of the two she was decribing. Both losses had
obviously deeply affected her, and although neither bereavement was
recent, for her they were a painful daily reality. She expressed considerable anger over her bereavement:

My husband – when he was alive – he used to do different
jobs for all of them; and my sister says, 'We don't half miss
old Art' – his name was Arthur, we called him Art … Oh,
the Almighty did take a good one there. He was
kind-hearted; he was clean. Everybody liked him. He was
well-liked, honest to God he was … The dirty, rotten,
stinking roughs that are allowed to live, standing on the
street corner, gambling, and things like that. The buggers are
allowed to live – that's what used to hurt me.

Sarah spoke with great vehemence and her eyes were full of tears as
she relived her pain. She was 'stuck' in the anger stage of her grief and
could not get out, nor was there counselling to help her.

Janet expressed her sense of hopelessness and resignation by
telling me how Green House for her was just a way 'to pass the time':

I've got to take things as they come. That's the only thing I
can do. I've lost my husband, you see, and there we are …
I've got to make the best of it, you see … Course, that was a
shock when I lost my husband. [Crying]

When I asked what was important for her now, she went on to tell of
her children, now both grown up, and both living in different parts of
the country – another kind of bereavement:

R.   ... so I don't see much of them.

I.   When you come here, what are the things about being here that you like?

R.   Well, I see what other people are doing, that's the only thing.

I.   Contact with other people – and that helps, does it?

R.   Yes, just a little bit.

Taken together, therefore, the importance of other people for clients, and the anguish, anger and despair engendered by their loss, would appear to mirror the picture of dementia as a dislocation of relationship that we shall see was also a feature of the carers' interviews: 'She doesn't recognise me' and 'She's not the person I used to know'. In other words, dementia was seen as a situation of mutual loss. The prevalence of ever-renewable grieving among clients with dementia not only indicated that their needs for help with their bereavement were not being met, but also perhaps was a pointer to a more generalised bereavement: the loss of meaningful and supportive relationships, brought about by the increasing communication difficulties produced by their dementia.

### Loss of home

Loss as a feature of interviews with clients in the in-patient facility perhaps reflected the fact of the ultimate loss of family, hearth and home which they had experienced. However, some of the day-hospital clients were already in residential or nursing homes, and so the subject also occurred in some day-hospital client interviews as well. After the loss of spouse and family, the loss of home could be the greatest deprivation eventually suffered by those with dementia. What does 'home' mean? Here is one of the best definintions that I know:

> A home exists where sentiment and space converge to afford attachment, stability, and a secure sense of personal control. It is an abiding place and a web of trustworthy connections, and anchor of identity and social life, the seat of intimacy

and trust from which we pursue our emotional and material needs. (Segal and Baumohl 1988, p.249)

It was interesting that the importance of one's own home was demonstrated in clients' interviews by its metaphorical use to indicate what was most needed and appreciated:

R. I enjoy the atmosphere of this place [Green House day-hospital].

I. The atmosphere.

R. The atmosphere is nice, very nice ... They are very nice people and the place is nice. You come 'home from home' – that's how I feel.

I. Home from home?

R. Home from home.

I. Nice thing to say.

R. Sounds very nice ... That's all I can – I can't say anything nicer than that. I look forward to coming.

I. You do?

R. I do. I look forward to coming. And I've met charming people here – just like coming home again.

So said Samuel of the day-hospital, where his care scores were consistently high and characterised by the greatest amount of his time being very positively coded in terms of personal interaction.

However, for another day-hospital attender, Mary, home ('my right home') was the place to which she was literally crying to be taken back. She attended Green House from a residential home, and she was in a wheelchair. She had therefore already lost her independence both in terms of mobility and of her own home. Mary did not like coming to Green House, because they had taken her shoes away and given her slippers to wear, so that she was afraid that she would have to stay there 'altogether'. She was evidently very nervous and afraid of those clients who wandered around or shouted out a lot, and particularly so of Daisy, the very aggressive woman day-hospital client who had been brought for respite care into the in-patient facility. This heightened Mary's unease, since she understood that those attending the day-hospital could find themselves taken into the in-patient area. The unsatisfactory nature of the building's design – the juxtaposition of the two different facilities within the same building – was clearly demonstrated in this case. It was possible for Mary to see through the large glass doors into the in-patient area, where not only did she see a more soporific environment and a more disturbed population, but from which she clearly feared that this aggressive fellow client would emerge – as indeed she often did. For Mary, then, Green House did not represent either 'a web of trust-worthy connections' or 'the seat of intimacy and trust'.

Yet for another day-hospital client, Charles, Green House was 'an anchorage'. Significantly, he attended Green House from his own home, where he was cared for by his wife. He was also aware of his condition (multi-infarct dementia). A strong and interesting person-ality, he had retained an extremely positive view of life and was able to accept the day-hospital as 'a prop'. He was still independent, both in his mobility and his living, and could therefore presumably afford to treat Green House as an additional support.

For Michael, in the in-patient unit, 'home' was the place he wished to get back to. Michael was the client noted for his 'escapes' from Green House, having been fetched back from the town centre on more than one occasion, and who had asked me if I could give him a lift home in my car ('I'm wondering how I could use you to drive me home'). Earlier in the interview he had repeated that there was 'nothing' he liked about being at Green House, saying:

> I'd rather be at home.

It would appear, therefore, that the Green House service was valued by those whose abilities were still relatively intact or who explicitly recognised that they needed 'a prop'. For these clients the Green House experience was very positive and 'home from home' was the highest accolade they could give it. However, for those who had lost their home – their 'real home' – and were separated from their loved ones ('I'd rather be at home because I have six grandchildren') Green House was definitely not perceived as 'home from home', but rather as somewhere from which they wished (and even tried!) to escape. The circularity of the problem was that precisely those clients whose confusional handicap was greater were the ones to lose what they most valued. From their testimonies it appeared that the supportive features of 'home' had not been transferred to Green House.

## Perspectives on dependence

There seemed to be three particular examples of the ways in which clients referred to the experience of dependence, two of which were negative, and one positive. The first two concerned the prevalence of what I came to call 'the parental analogy' when discussing their experience of Green House, and the second the awareness in one instance of detention under Mental Health Act section. The third, and positive, allusion to dependence came from a client who expressed great satisfaction with the physical care she received.

To begin with the parental analogy: as we have seen, it was an interesting feature of several client interviews that, when invited to talk about their experience of Green House, many of them recounted memory-stories involving their parents. There were various possible interpretations of this. One explanation could be the greater availability of older, long-term memories. Whereas more recent memories were fragmenting, memories of childhood remained, relatively speaking, clearer. Another explanation has been explored in Miesen's work on 'attachment theory and dementia' (Jones and Miesen 1992). However, as described in Chapter Two, the research method I used was to focus on the metaphorical content of such memory-stories.

There are, of course, other memories of childhood than those involving parents. So the question could be asked: why were these particular memories being recalled and recounted in this particular situation? All the client interviews took place actually in Green House. Also, the conversation always began with the same question: 'What is it like for you here, in Green House?' So it seemed legitimate, therefore, to infer that the situation of dependence in which these clients again found themselves could be resuscitating other memories of dependence from childhood. By analogy, then, the staff would be perceived in a parental role.

If this was the case it is perhaps a little disturbing that these memories seemed sometimes to be of strictness and lack of understanding. One in-patient respondent was concerned that any suggestions should be 'acceptable.' For example, he thought more use of the garden would be a good idea. He went on to refer to 'strict observance of any of these restrictions':

> I believe that they are pretty strict now ... Well, looking at it from my point of view, I would think that even I would have to be rather strict, otherwise if you overstep the mark at all, you quite properly would be ... I was saying – well, I mean, they could quite properly turn round and say, 'We can't agree to your coming in and around these parts and we shall have to cut down on them,' and I don't know exactly how fast they do come in when they do come.

Another client brought up parental memories of anger and violence – specifically, a physically abusive father. This was Sarah, who was still 'stuck' in the anger stage of grieving for her dead husband. She admitted that she attended Green House 'to get away from four walls ... I don't like to be on me own', having lived all her life within a large (and sometimes tempestuous) family. She said that she liked coming to Green House, but in the next breath acknowledged the dependent relationship:

> Everybody's kind. Nobody's rude to one another – mind you, if you were rude – don't have to be rude when people's looking after you.

This led her into an extended account of her (and her family's) relationship with her sometimes violent father:

> Oh, yes – it used to be terrible when we was younger ... He used to be spiteful to my Mum an' all – I've seen my Mum with many a black eye as a kid, and that all kept in your

memory, you know, all that sort of thing. It did mine anyway. Me and my sisters, we used to sit and cry to one another about it. 'What can we do?' we used to say. My sister was two years older than me. 'We can't do anything' ... I used to run away.

These memory stories need not be interpreted as Sarah's actually experiencing physical attack by staff. Indeed, her care scores in the DCM observations indicated that she was receiving a 'good' experience of care. It was more likely that the memories were indicative of the remembered levels of fear, anxiety, and impotent rage that she experienced as a child, and was now again experiencing as life withdrew from her spouse, home, and faculties, leaving her dependent on the care of others. For her, then, dependence was experienced not as stigmatising and a blow to self-respect, but as frightening.

Another example of how dependence could be perceived by clients concerned 'sectioning' under the Mental Health Act. This constituted a formal and legal recognition of a person's lack of fitness to control their own life, and the necessity of their dependence on qualified care. Given that the reason for admitting someone under Mental Health Act section was that they were incapable of understanding what was necessary for their own safety, it was interesting that James was interviewed precisely on the day that he was admitted under section. In our interview he clearly indicated his awareness (in his own terms) of the fact that he was now compulsorily detained, as together we searched for his hat. After explaining how he had been told he could no longer travel without a license, he continued:

I don't know where it is I want to go now, but I don't know which way to go. No, I don't. But if they know, they won't tell you. Because – I don't know if you know that – that's a secret part right along there.

His confidential manner and the way he nodded towards the staffroom indicated his awareness of the fact that staff had come to some kind of decision affecting his mobility to which he was not fully party. All he knew was that he could not 'travel' anymore. Yet this was all he wanted to do:

> Means a lot to me. I got to go back – I haven't been home for I don't know how long.

In other words, Green House did not feel like a refuge – or even an 'anchorage' – for this client, whose independence had been completely compromised.

However, for at least one client I interviewed, dependence was viewed positively, due, it would seem, to positive older associations of such a role at school. Rather than a parental analogy, therefore, Anna's memory seemed to be drawing an insitutional analogy with her experience of school. A school is an institution, and so this could also be interpreted as an implicit recognition of Green House as 'institutional'. Nevertheless, this was a testimony to the importance of the physical care delivered by the Green House service:

I.   Do you like coming here?

R.   Yeh, they are all very nice – give me a bath once a week.

I.   They give you a bath.

R.   Yeh, it's awful down my place, y'see. I can't get in it, not now – and she's got a moveable chair, moves up and down – electric.

I.   Here?

R.   Yes.

I.   And that's easier for you?

R.   Puts you in the bath and you don't hurt yourself.

I.   Yourself? Oh, your shoulder – yes, because you have a poorly shoulder.

R.   Yes.

I.   Do you like having a bath up here then?

R.   Yes – I got a bath at home, but I couldn't get in it and out of it on my own. Where here the nurse –

I.    – helps you?

R.    Yes, she do put me in electric chair, puts me up over the bath. It's a good thing, really, because I couldn't get in the bath.

Anna found talking about Green House brought up memories of being cared for and protected by her teachers at school. She had evidently been a sickly child and subject to bullying. The school doctor had explained to the teachers that they must not expect too much from her, and that they must protect her from the cruelty of the other children. The analogy would appear to be with the doctor at Green House, who had explained to staff that she was poorly and must be helped and protected – which she was very grateful that they did.

Anna was considered to be still only in an early 'stage' of dementia. Her own main preoccupation was with her incapacitated arm. She told me that her daughter lived opposite her and came in every day. So she was one of the clients who still retained much of the necessary supports in her life, apart from the day-hospital. For her, Green House provided an extra place of support and refuge. Her DCM care score indicated that she was receiving a 'good' (almost 'very good') experience of care. And this agreed with her own assessment of her experience.

In summary, therefore, it appeared that many clients recognised the state of the dependence in which they found themselves at Green House. They were aware of it, but brought to it their former analogous experiences from earlier in their lives. Inevitably, then, the experience of dependence in the present was individually variable, according to the quality and nature of those previous experiences for any given individual. Hence strictness, or the fear and impotent rage of an abusive parental relationship, were resuscitated for one, while for another the help and protection of kindly teachers and the school doctor informed her appreciation of supportive physical care. The Green House service was, therefore, inevitably the unwitting heir of former critical experiences of the dependent role.

*Interdependence*

Yet it was not only gratitude for necessary physical care that prompted clients to express their appreciation. Several respondents commented on the kindness of staff, and it was clear from the way that they did so that this was a genuine response and not mere politeness. Edna, who was in for respite care, referred to staff as 'people who give their services'. She continued by saying 'I think it is very important that we should mix with one another and … learn to appreciate what other people do for us, and give up – especially when they give up, err, spare time.' A former headmistress, she added her own evaluation of Green House: 'I think it runs on pretty good lines.'

Charles, in the day-hospital, found another way of referring to the staff: as 'teenagers' – thus defining them by the age difference. Age was seen by several of the clients I interviewed as the reason for their forgetfulness and for their need to be at Green House. Hence the description of the staff as teenagers – those who have their youth and strength:

I. The teenagers – what about the teenagers?

R. Oh, I reckon they're great. They've got everything going, haven't they?

I. They have.

R. Yes, yes.

I. You think they've got a lot going for them?

R. Oh, yes. 'Cos teenagers are just in that lovely age group what-have-you, and they can be ever so helping.

The point being made here was that those who still had their youth and strength were using it for the benefit of those who needed it. Charles suffered from multi-infarct dementia, and was interviewed on his first day back at the day-hospital after a serious stroke. He had clearly been shaken by this experience, but he had made a good recovery and returned to Green House looking physically frail but still very alert and cheerful. His wife had insisted that he be kept informed of his condition and be involved in all discussions and decisions about his care, so he knew that he suffered from a dementing illness.

Yet his attitude to life was remarkably positive, and his optimistic and generous philosophy of life was all the more impressive, coming as it did from one who was knowingly facing what for most people is an unimaginable abyss. His point was that experience had taught him that the help of others was what could bring one through those situations from which there may seem no way out:

R. Yes, I've been in places where you think to yourself: 'Well, I'm finished. Don't know what to do, don't know where to start!' And all that. Then something pops up – could be only a tu'penny-ha'penny little thing, but – you feel as though – it feels really that you've got a prop there really but you can't see the prop. Know what I mean?

I. An invisible prop?

R. Yeh, yeh! I think it's nice that – having peoples and that, to help. 'Cos often they can help. Yeh, I've got in positions where I've been in an awful state and then – come out lovely!

I. Because people helped you?

R. Yes, more than anything.

Earlier in the interview he had said:

R. I love it here.

I. You do?

R. Yes, because it's an anchorage.

I. An anchorage?

R. You know, not because you've got to lean completely on it, not because you've got to completely lean on, no ...

I. ... What exactly did you mean by an anchorage? Can you tell me a bit more about that?

R. You've got to have a little bit of prop.

I. A prop?

R.  Yeh. I find that – it's lovely. Lovely someone in the distance, probably, who could be good –

I.  So it's knowing there's someone if you need them?

R.  That's right. Yeh. It isn't putting on a person so much that they can be burdened, no, no. You've got to be self-supporting as well, yourself, haven't you, partially?

I.  That's right, yes you do. So you're saying that you like to be self-supporting but it's nice to know there's someone there if you need them.

R.  That's right, yes, yes.

I.  So Green House, for you, it's nice because you know it's here if you –

R.  That's right, yes. I love that. That's right. I'm not leaning on nobody, but you know there's somebody there if you want it. Because we all think really that we're so self-satisfied or what-have-you that we can do it all ourselves. But we can't – no, we can't. Many and many a day I find that you want the prop.

While Charles was expressing his deep appreciation of the support ('the prop') that the Green House staff provided, he was also keen to underline both his need and his ability to be 'self-supporting'. He was at pains at various points in the interview to emphasise that 'people are intelligent, resourceful':

> Because most people, you know, I expect you find, are so bright. People are brighter than we think ... give them half a chance, they can be resourceful, they can be helpful.

This was a clear plea to not be underestimated. While Charles 'loved' knowing that his 'anchorage' was there if he needed it, that did not of itself mean that he was therefore inferior. The fact that we could all need help and support from time to time in our lives did not justify a patronising attitude or an unequal relationship:

> You don't have to bend down on people, not that at all, no. It's give and take. Yes, I love that – give and take.

Significantly, Samuel had begun his interview by stressing the importance of people, and continued immediately to expatiate on why they were important. People are important because we all need each other:

R. People that make life worth living.

I. It is.

R. We all rely on one another, you know.

I. ... We do.

R. Everyone, everybody, he thinks he doesn't. He thinks he can manage with the car. But you've got to rely on people. Just like the chicken crossing the road [laughter]. Got to get to the other side!

Samuel went on to give an example of his own need to rely on the staff who collected him in 'the waggon' (the minibus) to take him to Green House. They had to check that he had turned the gas out and locked the door, because he admitted he was forgetful. He then launched into a series of autobiographical stories, whereby he constructed a vivid picture of himself as venerable craftsman, musician, father. In other words, he felt the need to establish a strong and worthy identity as a counterbalance for present frailty.

It was clear that from both his father and his 'boss' Samuel had acquired a very clearly gendered value system. He recounted the story of how, during the First World War, men who looked as if they were of an age and state of health to be in the army but were walking around in civilian clothes were accosted in the streets by women who pinned the badge of cowardice on them – a white feather. This had happened to his father – a strict and uncompromising man. Significantly, Samuel said of his father that:

> he was a very active man, looked younger than his age ...
> and he got this white feather.

Samuel himself was remarkably active for someone approaching his ninetieth year, and although he had white hair, he certainly did not look his age. He was being cared for by his daughter at home, and by a largely female care staff at Green House. It would seem that this dependence on women could be being interpreted by Samuel as inherently demeaning. Here again the present care relationship was coloured by previous life experiences and the values and feelings they created.

Interestingly Samuel spent much of the interview resting his hands on his stick. A stick can be seen symbolically as both the evidence of frailty and the symbol of dependence, or reliance. 'Stick' in everyday language, after all, belongs in the same category as 'crutch' – that on which a person leans for support and which enables him to walk. His eyes also rested often upon it, and he invited me to look at it too:

> That stick, that was given to one of my brothers for his leg.
> They all [his brothers] got wounded legs and they all got
> sticks, hobbling about on sticks. They were fine young
> fellows before they went into the army [in the First World
> War]. It killed a lot and it crippled a lot, a lot mentally too. It
> played hell with people, with the younger generation at that
> time. I can only use two words: 'played hell'. I can't say
> anything else.

Samuel was obliged to rely on his stick, but also on more than that, for he was dependent on others in matters practical as well as for sympathetic listening and understanding. He himself acknowledged:

> That stick's got a story!

The stick was like Samuel himself, the survivor of a long and colourful life, the bearer of memories of a bygone era. Samuel loved his stick, but to contemplate it also made him sad. Similarly he loved his daughter, and coming to Green House day-hospital; but his dependent status also made him uneasy. His wonderful memory-stories were his way of asserting his self-worth – in his own eyes as well as others'.

And he did not lose the opportunity during the interview of clarifying that he himself had known what it was to have to be responsible for someone and look after them; in his case, it had been his mother. He had wanted to go to work in France for a famous manufacturer of musical instruments there. When the opportunity came, however, he had had to turn it down because of his mother:

> They wanted me to work for them. But, you see, I had a widowed mother. I had brothers as well, but I like to play my part and be with my mother ... But I would have loved to have gone ... Always regretted it.

In other words, he wanted to demonstrate that he also understood the cost of caring and sometimes the extent of sacrifice involved. 'We all rely on one another,' he had said.

Pat, in the day-hospital, also expressed this desire for a more reciprocal care relationship. She had been a busy housewife, mother and grandmother – a farmer's wife – and now was nonplussed by all the time, peace and quiet on her hands. It seemed that her great desire was to be useful. To be the recipient of the care and good labours of others was an unaccustomed state, and clearly challenged her whole sense of identity:

I. I noticed that you were in the group this morning making fruit salad.

R. Oh yes, whatever they had to do.

I. Do you enjoy the things?

R. Yes, I do. They want to put it out for me to – well, do what they are doing. I don't mind being there to help them out with anything. Yes, it's quite good really.

I. Any other activities that you like to do here?

R. I don't know of anything. I don't mind doing like I'm doing now or little jobs there are, you know. They want to get things done and I'm quite willing to do a bit towards it.

I. So you enjoy being able to help?

R. Yes, oh yes. Yes, if they want it done, I'm quite willing to put up with anything, yes.

I. Putting up with anything?

R. Yes, well –

I.   Is that how it seems?

R.   Err, I suppose so, really. Anything they want done or doing and might want a bit of help, I'm quite willing to stand by … If they want some help and they asked for it, I'd be quite willing to have a go at doing whatever they might want some help with. I don't have much in that way.

It seemed to me that some of the clients spoke with the wisdom of those who have already passed beyond a barrier of confusion, fear and suffering which separated them forever from the way those behind them saw the world. There was a genuine appreciation of the fact that they (like all of us) need help and care, and there was also a recognition of the cost that this can entail to the giver. They reminded me gently that there was also a cost to the receiver of care, and that this can be mitigated if only we could understand that care and support have to be reciprocal. Charles seemed to sum it up:

I think as we are individually we can be very weak. We might think we can take it all on – on ourselves. You can't now. It's bigger than that.

## Conclusion

These were only 22 interviews, but they represented about two-thirds of all the clients using the Green House service at that time. And they covered individuals across a wide range of handicap, from the merely rather forgetful, through the increasingly confused and agitated, to those who were no longer considered able to function in their own homes and who were now 'in-patients' indefinitely. Yet their interviews showed remarkable patterns in terms of what was uppermost in their minds when asked about their experience of Green House. The most remarkable was the awareness demonstrated, not only of the interview situation, but of their own confusion and forgetfulness, and of their intimations of mortality. The significance of relationships with other people – for better or for worse – was often the first thing that they wished to talk about – and the subject to which they would return. The expression of feelings about losses – of faculties, loved ones, home, and role in life – was a further moving testimony to the fact that dementia is not a state of waking anaesthesia. However comforting we might find it to believe that people with dementia do not really know what is happening to them, the clients I interviewed told a different story. Yet they lived with their awareness, for the most part accompanied by considerable tolerance and concern for those who cared for them – either relatives or professional staff. While these interviews highlighted the individual emotional and psychological 'luggage' which each person brought to their enforced dependency, they also contained invitations to a new way of framing the care relationship, so that it is not about passive receipt but a two-way, mutual process. Perhaps this is the key to finding ways of caring which do not exact such a cost in terms of self-esteem, identity, and psychological well-being. It really does pay to listen.

CHAPTER 5

# What the clients experienced

*From observing individual clients in their daily life at Green House using Dementia Care Mapping, a certain picture emerged of care delivered according to clients' ability levels.*

As well as interviewing the clients of Green House, I also spent a lot of time observing what happened in both the day-hospital and the in-patient unit. It was necessary to do both. For while I was, in fact, able to interview two-thirds of the clients, there remained others whose perspective I was not able to access. The great advantage of observing behaviour, and of reading it as meaningful communication, is that this is a method which does not rule out anyone. Whatever their verbal communication skills (or lack of them) all the clients of the service could be observed. And I also needed to explore 'on the ground' the issues which had arisen from the interviews. For if awareness, the significance of other people, loss and dependence were the major themes that emerged from my interviews with clients, how did these correlate with people's actual lived experience of care? In other words, what was the relationship between what seemed to be uppermost in clients' minds and the care that the Green House service provided for them?

As described in Chapter Two, Dementia Care Mapping (DCM) was the observational method I used. Analysing these DCM observations also provided some additional insights into clients' lived experience of care. (At this point I should point out that the DCM findings to which I shall refer reflect the method in its original form, as Tom, Kathy and I used it at that time. Since then certain evolutional changes in the method have taken place, but none of these would invalidate the findings quoted here.) While DCM constituted the framework for recording and measuring my observations, I also, of course, took copious field notes. I tried to record as much as possible of what I witnessed, both during and after interviews, and during and after mapping sessions. In fact, whenever I was around Green House for whatever reason, I developed the habit of noting down events that occurred, particularly those that related directly or indirectly to clients. Thus I acquired a fund of small narratives or vignettes of dementia care at Green House. These built up an enriched picture of clients' lived experience there, on which I shall draw in this chapter.

## Clients' awareness and their experience of care

In their interviews the clients of Green House had shown their awareness of their situation, their memory-problems, and many other things. Indeed, they were all clearly pleased by the recognition that they might have a perspective, which just being invited to give their views implied. But as we shall see, other people applied their own criteria to the question of client awareness. Most notably, the staff evaluated clients' awareness in terms of their ability to express themselves in words. Those with whom they could converse were deemed more aware, and those with whom they could not were deemed for the most part to be in a state of merciful oblivion. This continuum of awareness-judged-by-verbal-skills was reflected in the day-hospital and in-patient unit divide, and indeed, also in the service's terminology. A relatively more verbally skilled person was a client of the day-hospital. A less skilled one was a patient in the in-patient unit.

In view of the way in which awareness and verbal ability were thus confounded, therefore, one of the most interesting findings from the DCM observations was the correlation between verbal ability levels and measured levels of well-being and ill-being. Quite simply, the more able you were, the greater the level of well-being. That is, the more 'aware' you were considered to be, the greater the level of well-being you would experience in the care environment. Individual well-being is to a certain degree self-supported. But it is also much more rewarding for staff to work with relatively more able clients. This, of course, leads to a virtuous circle: those who are more able and feel better about themselves anyway, also receive more interactive care. However, sadly the opposite is also true. For there was also a vicious circle with regard to the less able, whose levels of ill-being were unaddressed by those around them, thus leading to further deterioration.

How did this picture of the relationship between clients' ability levels and their well-being emerge? The key lay precisely in the fact that, unlike the clients' interviews, DCM was not contingent on the client's ability to communicate verbally. As I was using DCM to 'map' the individual experience of all clients irrespective of their state of cognitive impairment or their verbal skills, I was able to divide them into four groups:

- those who attended the day-hospital and could be interviewed

- those who were in-patients and could be interviewed

- those who attended both facilities and could be interviewed

- those from both day-hospital and in-patient facility who could not be interviewed because their verbal skills were apparently non-existent.

I wanted to know what was the experience of care for clients in each of these groups. For instance, did clients in each group appear to have much the same experiences, or was there a characteristic profile for each group? In fact, the latter proved to be the case.

We can look at them in turn.

1. To begin with the day-hospital, all the clients I interviewed there had higher Individual Care Scores than those in the other groups. Indeed, the average care score for day-hospital clients put

them in the 'very good' category. Because in each time-frame DCM records both the activity or behaviour of the person and the level of well- or ill-being, it was possible to understand something of what contributed to these clients' overall 'very good' experience in the day-hospital.

Far and away the most significant factor proved to be social inter-action (A). This was the highest scoring Behaviour Category Code (BCC) for every client, and it was nearly always the one which had occupied the greatest amount of their time there. This meant that these day-hospital clients' most important experience of the care environment was interpersonal contact per se. This could be either with staff or with other clients. And because A is a code only allocated for interaction when *no* other activity is happening (such as eating or drinking, walking about, receiving physical care), this meant that the activity in which day-hospital clients spent most of their time, and which gave them their highest sense of well-being there (as judged by their behaviour and body language), was interpersonal interaction 'for the sake of it'.

However, it also emerged that games-like activities (G) supported some of the higher care scores of several clients in the day-hospital. In other words, where people's ability and personality allowed them to join in games (of cards, for instance), this provided a congenial context within which social interaction could (and did) occur. Of course, this type of activity was not to everyone's taste. Nevertheless, it shows that the importance of other people, of which so many of the clients had spoken in their interviews, was also a feature of their experience of the day-hospital. But it was so because their conversa-tional abilities allowed them to be considered 'aware'.

2. The overall average care score for all the *patients* in the in-patient unit was considerably lower: only towards the top of the 'fair' range of scores. In other words, their average experience of care was almost – but not quite – 'good'. Within this overall group, however, I went on to distinguish between those whom I had been able to interview, and those whom I had not. I should add that I interviewed pretty much

everyone who could still pronounce words – just as Laura had instructed me.

Looking first at those clients in the in-patient facility whom I had been able to interview, they had a higher average care score ('good') than that for the in-patient unit overall. Their greater ability to communicate meant that staff perceived them as more aware. In fact, the distribution of care scores in the in-patient facility clearly mirrored the distribution of remaining communication skills in the clients observed. This is the more striking because DCM is deliberately designed so that any client may receive as high a care score as any other, irrespective of their level of handicap. However, those clients with greater remaining social and communication skills had higher care scores. In other words, the care they experienced supported greater levels of well-being than those found in clients who did not speak. The latter remained in states of apathy, somnolence or sometimes continual distress for extensive periods. When Tom and I began to feed these results back to staff it did not appear to surprise them. They apparently accepted that this would be the case.

In fact, the greatest amount of time spent by each client in the in-patient area during the periods I observed was in sitting, just looking around (B). Even the slightest greeting, a smile or wave across the room, could automatically change the recording from 'passive involvement' (B) to 'social interaction' (A). So the DCM observations painted a picture of the in-patient area as a generally un-stimulating environment with far lower levels of personal interaction. As in the day-hospital, however, certain (more able, more 'aware') clients sometimes had higher care scores, boosted by games-like activity (G). For instance, I particularly remember an unusual session of gin rummy involving the occupational therapist and three clients (two of whom, Jane and Edna, were in for respite care), from which gales of laughter blew across the lounge, as each player rediscovered a talent for cheating – and an 'awareness' of this in each other! For some of these clients 'social interaction' in and of itself (A) also contributed to their positive scores. Another contributor was 'labour' (L), which refers to time-frames when the client was involved either in 'real' work, such as helping staff in some task, or in 'pseudo-work', where it appeared that the client was carrying out an activity which from their perspective might be seen as work – such as dusting, or moving chairs.

But the most significant boost to the Individual Care Scores of clients in the in-patient facility was eating and drinking (F). Mealtimes and the giving of food and drink generally appeared to belong to the best part of care in the in-patient unit. To test this I actually mapped a period there which did not include any mealtimes. The resulting comparison more than proved the point. From the overall average of 'fair–nearly-good' for the same clients in the other periods I observed, the average for this 'no meal' period fell to barely above the lowest DCM range of 'much improvement needed'! If you were considered 'less aware', the most positive support for your well-being in this care environment was likely to come only from ingesting food. That is, it seemed that these clients were accepted as physically present with physical needs, and not emotionally present or 'aware', with corresponding 'feeling' needs.

3. Four clients I interviewed attended both the day-hospital and sometimes also the in-patient unit for respite care. Their average care score dropped from when I mapped them in the day-hospital to those periods in the in-patient unit when they were admitted for respite care. In the day-hospital the average put them towards the top-of-the-range of 'good' care. But when they were admitted for respite care this dropped to very near the bottom of that range. So although they remained just within the 'good' range, clearly their experience of care in the day-hospital had been considerably better than that in the in-patient facility. Also, as with the other clients in the in-patient area, the prevalent activity was sitting just looking around (B), whereas it was social interaction (A) when they were in the day-hospital.

However, for one of them, Jane, the drop in average care score was slightly less. Most of my observations of her showed that when admitted for respite care she was still involved in a relatively good amount of 'social interaction' (A) and games-like activity (G) scores. She was still well able to communicate verbally, and was possessed of a strong personality which enabled her to initiate social contacts. Her reactions to people and events left no-one in any doubt as to her awareness! However, this could also work against her. The DCM method also records episodes of the 'malignant social psychology' which Tom identified as a critical part of the downward spiral of dementia (Kitwood 1990). Such episodes ('personal detractions') could be words or actions which would tend to undermine a person's sense of themselves as a valuable human being. Jane tended to receive quite a few of these 'personal detractions' while in the day-hospital, where her strength of character and occasional flashes of bad language were not always appreciated by the staff. This could result in her being rebuked, and even banished to sit in a corner of the day-hospital away from the rest of the group. It was as if her (recognised) awareness was expected to mean that she would behave in ways acceptable to staff; they found it difficult to cope with her contrariness, and sometimes behaved towards her in a punitive manner, which effectively used her awareness against her. For to be aware is to be aware of being punished. In the in-patient unit, however, staff perhaps had reduced expectations of people, and showed greater tolerance of her, and she seemed more relaxed there, and was even allowed to join in games of cards and some other group activities skilfully organised by the occupational therapist.

4. The final group were those whom I was not able to interview. There were four clients in the day-hospital and ten clients in the in-patient unit. I analysed their individual care scores separately.

One of them, Joy, was an exceptional case. Her husband did not wish that either he or she should be interviewed. In fact, Joy herself was very socially skilled and well able to communicate verbally. Her average care score was well within the 'very good' range. On each of the three occasions that she was observed, 'social interaction' (A) was the most common coding, as it was with the other day-hospital clients who had been able to be interviewed.

The other three day-hospital clients whom I did not interview were incapable of it because their language skills were almost non-existent. Their average Individual Care Score was 'good,' but considerably less than the 'very good' average care score for the day-hospital clients who *had* been able to be interviewed. And there was another difference. Rather than 'social interaction' (A) being the most frequently observed activity, the most common behaviours observed for these clients were sitting just looking around (B), eating and drinking (F), walking about (K), and sleep (N). One person, Daisy, in particular was *always* wandering, never still. Another, Una, who slept much of the time, I observed also had many episodes of 'unresponded to communication' (U). That is, she would reach out to someone who passed by, or call out softly, but no one replied. I also often observed her in states of distress (D), also unacknowledged. So was sleep Una's refuge from unresponsiveness and neglect? After all, even when she did try to initiate interaction, no one acknowledged it. And when she was clearly upset, no one attempted to alleviate her distress. Her subjective world could be understood as one not worth staying awake for. It seemed that her limited ability to communicate and interact, particularly verbally, had a critical effect on her experience of care, and this in turn led to more withdrawn behaviour.

Still lower was the average care score for the ten clients in the in-patient area whom I could not interview – down towards the middle of the 'fair' range. This was below average for the in-patient unit as a whole, and considerably lower than the average for those in-patients who were able to be interviewed (who had achieved 'good'). Among those clients whom I could not interview were some people with particularly low care scores, in fact well down in the lowest 'much improvement needed' range. Indeed, one client on one occasion actually had an individual care score of 0. But could we call this 'care'?

These very low-scoring clients – among them Joe from Chapter One – were the most inarticulate and withdrawn patients. While good attention was for the most part paid to their physical needs, with the exception of mealtimes and toileting routines they were largely left to their own devices for long periods of time, each of them inhabiting a chair, and a world, alone. Their most frequently recorded activities were eating and drinking, just sitting looking round, sleeping, and walking about. Usually the latter just meant movement between the living-room and the dining-room, or the living-room and the toilet.

A strong indicator of the unstimulating and soporific nature of the in-patient environment, a great deal of the time, was the fact that it was actually possible for me to 'map' between ten and fourteen clients on my own. Normally the detailed nature of the observations required means that it should only be possible for a single observer to map five or six clients at a time. However, with so little going on in the environment, mapping all the clients in the in-patient area together presented no problem. I could spend an hour or more merely writing down rows of N (sleep) or B (sitting looking around). In such circumstances N becomes quite a temptation for the mapper too!

In the next chapter we shall see how many of the staff respondents thought that client awareness was related to their interactional and communication skill levels, and that consequently different care styles were applied for the clients on either side of this divide. In fact, this different care culture could be measured by the quantitatively different experience of the care environment of the different groups of clients, reflecting their different levels of communication handicap. I have summarised this in Graph 1. For from the above four groups I was actually able to separate out seven in, as it were, descending order of ability. The most able were the day-hospital interviewees, then those who attended both day-hospital and in-patient area for respite care. Then came the in-patient facility interviewees, followed by the day-hospital clients who could not speak and so were not interviewed. Surprisingly, the day-hospital-and-respite-care interviewees scored even lower than the day-hospital clients who could not be interviewed when they were admitted to the in-patient area; the more lively and sociable environment of the day-hospital clearly ensured that even those who could not communicate there still received a better experience of care than those who *could* still communicate verbally when they were admitted for respite care. This was for them, therefore, a respite from better levels of well-being! They still fared better than the overall average for clients in the in-patient area, however. And finally, those with the lowest experience of well-being were those in the in-patient area who could not speak.

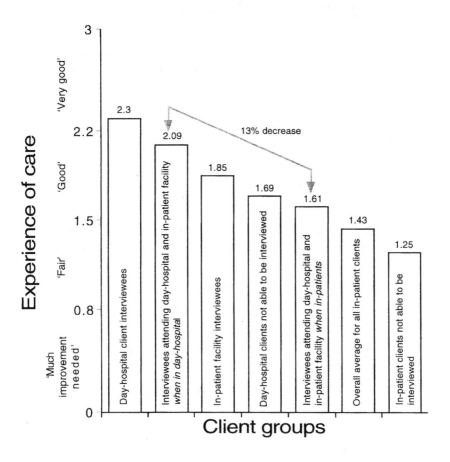

*A comparison of the care experience of client groups differing in verbal communication skills.*

So we can see that the greater the handicap, the less good the experience of care. And the mediating factor was the staff's belief that awareness could be judged by verbal ability. Where it was judged to be absent, even such 'awareness' as looking around one, reaching out to a passer-by, or showing distress went unacknowledged. People do not see what they do not expect to see. In this way staff were seemingly unaware of the awareness of their clients, so that the most needy clients received the least support for their personhood as measured by their levels of well-being.

## Clients' experience of social contact or isolation

Sometimes what we might call this lack of awareness on the part of people *without* dementia meant that good things in the Green House service went unrecognised. For instance, we have seen from the interviews how much clients valued the congenial company of other people in the day-hospital. Clearly, addressing needs does not necessarily depend on recognizing them, since it is possible that people's needs may be met, as it were, coincidentally – that is, without their having been part of the motivation or action plan of the doer. This, indeed, would appear to explain the phenomenon of the daily transport to the day-hospital.

Three of the day-hospital clients mentioned their journeys to and from Green House in the minibus – 'the waggon' as Samuel referred to it. For all of them this seemed to be a positive experience. As Green House served a rural area, clients often spent considerable time travelling to and from it in the minibus. Both staff and managers often voiced concern over this. Transport was seen, particularly by the staff, as taking up time that could more valuably ('therapeutically') be spent actually in the day-hospital.

Yet the clients themselves viewed the minibus experience as a particularly positive one. Indeed, as I observed them I came to think of these expeditions as 'transports of delight'! Someone came to fetch and welcome them, and then conscientiously took them back home and settled them in again. This was clearly an important feature of the Green House experience for them.

Significantly, the care scores for clients during their journeys in the minibus were very high – averaging 'very good'. This put the time spent on the minibus as among the very best times that clients enjoyed from the Green House service, and it appeared to bear out the clients' own testimony that journeys to and from Green House day-hospital were an important and positive experience for them. In fact, there were no negative references to transport in any of the client interviews. Indeed, several clients explicitly expressed a desire to go out and about more! One day-hospital client, Doris, repeatedly mentioned her love of walking, and even said she would enjoy going swimming. And Norma, in the in-patient unit, after telling me she had been in Green House for 'a very, very, very long time', said:

> I do like to go places – the car.

From the moment the minibus arrived, each client received a very personalised service. They were greeted by name, with inquiries about themselves, their families, or their homes, thus reinforcing their sense of identity. They also received quality physical care in helping them get ready for the journey, and onto the minibus. During the journey they were in a confined space, which naturally intensified the amount of personal interaction; it was not possible for anyone to be 'left out' in such intimate circumstances. Many clients showed evident delight as they greeted and made room for each other. The journey itself was obviously interesting to many of them – it being possibly the only time they were able to re-establish contact with the outside world. Arrival at Green House was the occasion for more physical care as people were helped off the minibus, and greeted by the rest of the day-hospital staff coming out to arm them down the little garden path into the day-hospital area. The welcoming cup of tea or coffee rounded off this whole episode with warmth and satisfaction. Yet, sadly, no one apart from the clients seemed to be aware of the value of these transport experiences.

We have already seen (Graph 1) that the day-hospital clients did, indeed, have a far better, and more social, experience of care than those in the in-patient area. Their average care score was 'very good', rising to an even higher average in the minibus. And in terms of their valuing the friendly company of others, a profile of their activities there showed that social interaction (A) was their most often recorded activity. So observation bore out the evidence from the clients' interviews: Green House provided them with a positive social experience – and that is what they said they appreciated so much.

The second most frequently recorded activity was eating and drinking (F), which was also a very sociable activity, conducted round small tables, with care being taken to seat people with those with whom they were especially friendly. I was told that the earlier practice of staff and clients all lunching together had been discontinued due to the organisation's new ruling about staff meals. Most of the staff regretted losing the 'normality' of the former way of doing things, but tried to compensate by sitting down with clients when they had finished serving.

However, whereas both staff and carers in their interviews spoke of the importance of 'stimulation', observation showed another picture. First, despite the high levels of interaction, the third most recorded activity even in the day-hospital was sitting just looking around (B). Second, the total amount of time spent in activities such as handicrafts (H), watching television or reading magazines (M), work or 'pseudo-work' (L), games (G), intellectual activity such as quizzes (I) and physical exercise (J), when counted all together, was still less than the fourth most recorded activity: walking about (K). Hence it seemed that staff's concern with stimulation was not translated into a great deal of structured 'activities'. The high care scores were the result of companionship per se: both that of clients with staff, and among the clients themselves.

There were, however, some negative experiences of social contact even in the day-hospital. The tearful anxiety of Mary, whose shoes had been exchanged for slippers, and who was in perpetual fear of being accosted by the 'wandering' Daisy, has already been described. Una, who attended the day-hospital from a nearby nursing home, was very confused indeed in her speech, and her interview in fact represented the limit of what could be achieved using the particular 'depth' interviewing technique. She wandered the day-hospital, mostly alone, in greater or lesser degrees of confusion and anxiety. She was unable and unwilling for the most part to join in any structured activities, and her verbal difficulties meant that she did not have much in the way of social interaction. That is, one-to-one conversations between her and other clients were non-existent, and with staff they were infrequent.

The same was often true of another day-hospital client, Vic, who was not only confused, but also almost blind and deaf as well. I had considered that it would not be possible to interview him – possibly incorrectly. One of the staff was particularly fond of him, and when she was on duty she would spend much time physically reassuring him by just sitting with him, holding hands or arm-in-arm. One afternoon, to everyone's astonishment, this companionship remarkably enabled him to join in singing an old song with the other clients – just for a moment. However, much of his time was spent more or less isolated (although physically in the group), calling for his daughter, with whom he lived.

Those day-hospital clients whom I could not interview also averaged lower care scores: 'good' compared with the overall average care score for the day-hospital of 'very good'. Their most common activities were just sitting looking about (B), followed by eating and drinking (F), walking about (K), and sleeping (N). The client who also spent a great deal of her time asleep (unusual in the day-hospital) and had several 'unresponded to communication' (U) episodes, was similar in her behaviour to the very handicapped clients in the in-patient area. But it was different – and more poignant – in that she was reaching out for companionship in a sociable environment, and still was not answered.

Such isolation was much more generally noticeable in the in-patient area, where each client seemed to live in a world of their own. The average care score for the in-patient area was only 'fair' (compared with 'very good' in the day-hospital). The most commonly recorded activity was just sitting looking round (B), in the same way as it was for the clients who could not be interviewed in the day-hospital. Just as for them, too, eating and drinking (F) was the most prominent positive feature of their care experience. It seemed that, in default of verbal interaction, food and drink became staff's preferred medium of care. That is, through the giving of food, often with much (or even total) physical assistance required, staff were able to provide the meaningful turn-taking and gestures of affection and concern that were otherwise denied many of these clients. The context of the giving and receiving of physical nourishment constituted the optimum experience of social interaction for the most handicapped clients, and perhaps also the most satisfying professional one for staff, as they could see they had something to give that was needed and valued, and could watch it being accepted.

In fact, interpersonal contact for these clients was usually only with members of staff, rather than with each other. However, Norma and Mildred, two of the women clients in the in-patient area, were the exception to this rule, and had a habit of sitting together. They would doze together side by side on the sofa, the smaller one resting her head on the taller one's shoulder. Overall, though, the lack of resident interaction in the in-patient area, as opposed to the day-hospital, was very notable.

But when certain staff members were on duty (notably one very experienced unqualified nurse and an occupational therapist) this could change temporarily, and then there would be small group activities, such as playing cards or brass-polishing, which were obviously enjoyed by all concerned and which also led to one-to-one interaction between residents. Mealtimes also could then become very different. As clients were treated with greater respect and sensitivity they also began to consider each other and each other's needs.

For instance, one Saturday evening Tom and Kathy and I measured an interesting and unusual increase in the care scores for all the clients in the in-patient unit, even though the actual number of staff on duty was less than there had been during the day. Then there had been four staff (two qualified and two unqualified) caring for fifteen clients.

That evening there were two unqualified staff caring for fourteen patients, while the qualified member of staff (who was an agency nurse) 'specialed' one very sick client in her room. Since DCM is only used in communal settings, it was the experience of the fourteen clients in the living-room and dining-room areas that we mapped. The average care score jumped from 'fair' to 'good', a very significant positive increase in the average experience of care delivered to the same clients in the same environment – but by different staff – over consecutive shifts. And the process by which this was achieved was particularly interesting with reference to the question of individual clients' sense of isolation.

The two unqualified staff were each new to dementia care: one had had many years experience in 'geriatric' nursing, and the other was a young student nurse gaining experience by 'bank' working. (The 'bank' was a method for sharing staff flexibly across different sites, so that staff shortages could be compensated for without having to rely so heavily on outside agency staff, who did not know the clients or the environment.) Both these staff approached their clients in a particularly respectful, imaginative and genuinely caring manner. The feelings, wishes and dignity of each client were conscientiously respected in every instance observed. The effect of this on the whole atmosphere of the environment meant that clients benefited doubly, for they began to interrelate among themselves in caring and positive ways, and thereby contributed to each other's experience of being cared for, by caring for each other.

One example of this occurred during the evening meal. Norma and Mildred, who often sat and snoozed together in the living-room, were seated at a table together. Mildred (who no longer used language) had a habit of playing with the cutlery and dropping it on the floor, and so her place had not been laid, although her friend's had been – as had everybody else's. It was staff's practice only to give Mildred her cutlery with her food. Norma was still able to find some words. She was the client who, in her interview, had said: 'I need to be me!' Her concern now was for her friend's identity (and status). She began to show signs of agitation and distress, calling to the staff.

The student nurse came over and sat beside her, giving her his full attention, and began to understand from her gestures and phrases that she did not like to have her own place laid, but not her friend's. This was offensive to her. He explained gently why the staff had been told not to provide Mildred with cutlery until the plate of food was also on the table, but this was clearly not a satisfactory reply. So he checked with Norma that she really did want her friend's place to be laid – even given that she might throw all the cutlery on the floor. She nodded assent. So he agreed, and brought over the cutlery and laid the place for her friend – who was able to stop her incessant nodding and table-cleaning movements for long enough to give her champion a little smile. The cutlery remained on the table untouched, until her plate of food arrived, when she used it appropriately.

Norma was obviously calmer and pleased with the results of her intervention. She had not only the pleasure of seeing her friend treated in the same way as herself, but the great satisfaction of having been the instrument of that happening. She sat very erect for the rest of the mealtime, glancing over at her friend from time to time with a smile of affection and pride. They had both achieved something. They had both been *enabled* to achieve something. Several of the other clients in the dining-room were interacting in analogous fashion – passing things to each other, smiling and nodding at each other, and exchanging a few words if they were able to speak.

The quality of interpersonal interaction between clients had been clearly affected by the manner of care delivery. Since care was being given to individual clients on an equal, respectful and trusting basis, the individual clients were enabled to value one another also. Individual clients' sense of isolation and 'not belonging' had evidently been lessened. This was all the more interesting given that it was noticeable in the in-patient area how individual clients often appeared to find the presence of other clients disturbing and even frightening.

In summary, observation showed that the benefits of congenial companionship and friendly interaction, which client respondents had said they valued, were available to those whose handicaps were relatively fewer, particularly with regard to verbal communication skills. Graph 1 is again pertinent here. It shows clearly how clients' positive experience of care, as measured by DCM in terms of their well-being, deteriorates with the deterioration of their verbal communication skills. Interestingly, the day-hospital clients who were not capable of being interviewed still received a higher care score than those clients who could be interviewed who were in the in-patient area for respite care. The overall atmosphere of the day-hospital was livelier, the staffing ratio usually more favourable. So even verbally uncommunicative clients still received more interaction (companionship) than did those who could still communicate in the relatively much less sociable environment of the in-patient facility.

## Did the Green House service address clients' sense of loss?

And what clues could the DCM observations offer about establishing whether clients' preoccupations with regard to loss were actually being met? We have seen that the more able clients (largely those attending the day-hospital), especially those who explicitly recognised their problems, found Green House 'home from home' and 'an anchorage'. For Samuel, for example, Green House was 'home from home' because it provided him with the congenial company he needed, which was not available at home because his wife had died and his daughter was out at work all day. His care scores were consistently towards the top-of-the-range of 'very good'. Social interaction (A) was his most frequently recorded activity. The loss of familiar company was therefore clearly being compensated for, and Samuel was measurably in receipt of 'very good' care.

For Charles the same situation applied. His understanding of his condition additionally led him to describe Green House as 'an invisible prop' – a support that was there when you needed it, and the awareness of its existence was very reassuring. Fortified by this, Charles could afford to be open to the good things life still offered from time to time. It was he who, one sunny spring afternoon, travelling through the local countryside in the minibus, rejoiced at seeing all the daffodils in the familiar country lanes by reminiscing about the places he saw, and then singing several old music-hall songs at the top of his voice, his face wreathed in smiles, and nodding a benediction to all who caught his eye.

For these clients, however, the loss of faculties was relatively less advanced, and the loss of home not even on the horizon. Both were cared for by their next of kin in their own home. For this particular sub-group, then, Green House was providing very much what they needed.

Yet what of those day-hospital clients who had spoken of their loss of loved ones – their grief? Jane, who had spoken so angrily about the loss of her much loved husband, still retained her communication skills, but lived alone at home. Her bereavements, therefore, were a matter of everyday experience, since she got up to an empty house and went to bed in it each night. She used her interview to talk in detail of both her dead father and her dead husband. She spoke with great vehemence, and her eyes were full of tears as she relived her pain.

After the interview one of the qualified nurses came over to speak with her, and she continued to speak of her dead husband and father in the same distressed vein – although at the same time she referred to them as if they were still alive and waiting for her at home. The nurse gently reminded her of what year it was and of her own age, and followed this up by trying to get her to understand that it was therefore unlikely that her father would be at home waiting for her to come home for tea. From tearful distress her face changed to a look of blank confusion. Eventually she said: 'I'll have to think about that.' She remained unusually quiet and introspective for the rest of the afternoon.

Such reminders of so-called present reality were not uncommon, as staff seemed to have understood 'reality orientation' in this way. Also they had a compassionate desire to remove someone from the distress of former pain. However, such responses not only devalued the acute nature of the revived feelings of grief and loss, but also increased the client's confusion, as to pain was added incomprehension and the fear of their own muddled thought processes. Since, as we have seen, many of the Green House client respondents were aware of their confusion, such mishandling of their grieving must have undermined even further their fragmenting self-esteem. It was also a statement of inequality on the part of staff: as if 'reality' could only be that perceived by themselves.

Although Jane was one of the 'high scorers' in terms of care scores, and although for her, too, social interaction (A) was the most frequently recorded activity, her need for help with the anger and denial of her grieving went unrecognised and unmet. The validity of the subjective reality of every individual requires recognition in dementia care environments, so that a client's identity and self-respect are protected. If a client is living the pain of grief now, then that is *their* present reality, and their need is for help and support with that.

As for the clients in the in-patient unit who had, by definition, already suffered the definitive loss of home (and this because of their already far greater loss of faculties), what was their experience? As we have seen, the average care score for this client group was far lower and their most commonly recorded activity was sitting looking round (B). That is, they spent most of their time just sitting and watching the environment with no great show of alertness or enthusiasm. They were awake and aware – but that was all.

Here again, therefore, the double standard applied. For those whose losses were relatively less, the service provided a better answer to need. For those whose losses were far greater, the response to need was far less than adequate. Indeed, when I constructed a profile of all the 'care values' recorded (Graph 3, p.187), I saw that nearly half of all the in-patient clients' time during the periods I observed was spent at only the 'maintenance care' (+1) level. ('Maintenance care' is where there is an absence of signs of ill-being, but nothing more positive than that.) For the most part, then, these clients sat alone among familiar strangers, devoid of companionship, and withdrawn into a solitary world from which no hand drew them back into the warmth of interaction. It would be hard not to interpret their presence at Green House as yet another loss.

Those who could do so wandered living-room and corridors in seemingly perpetual search. What they were seeking was not often clear, yet it represented physically the feelings of loss so many of them referred to in their different ways. One in-patient client, David, who came in often for 'respite' care, created tension by continually walking around whistling for his dog. Ostensibly it was the noise which annoyed. But beyond that I felt that it highlighted the fact that clients were experiencing feelings of loss beyond most of our abilities to imagine – and staff were experiencing their own feelings of power-lessness to answer those needs. Even to recognise them perhaps was too threatening. The whistling never stopped.

## Clients' experience of dependence

It is, of course, important to remember that the experience of dependence is not necessarily of itself related to handicap as perceived by others. Indeed, the experience of dependence referred to in some of the client interviews was an internal (and therefore in itself unobservable) mental state or subjective feeling.

Of course, with regard to clients' actual daily experience of dependence in Green House we have already looked at the fact that the quality of clients' experience of care correlated directly with their level of ability or handicap – particularly in regard to verbal communication skills. The greater the handicap, the less good the experience of care was seen to be (see Graph 1). However, the particular relevance here is that the more handicapped the client, the greater his or her dependence on the care of others. Therefore, there would appear to be a relationship between individual client dependency levels as indicated by their level of handicap, and the experience of care. The staff, managers and carers in their interviews all indicated that the level of handicap was interpreted in terms of 'awareness' and 'insight'. The implication here was that, with increasing handicap, the motivation for care changed from an identification with the suffering and frustration of a recognised fellow human being, to the compassionate practice towards those perceived to be in a 'vegetative state', arising from a need to preserve the caregiver's (and the service's) self-image as humane. And as this motivation changed, so did the relationship with the individual clients. It seemed, therefore, that the increase in handicap, which led to an increase in dependency, in turn led to a decrease in the quality of care experienced.

Yet observation showed that the amount of time spent by clients in receiving 'practical, personal physical care' (P) in the communal environment of the in-patient unit registered only on average 2.5 per cent of the total time mapped. It is, of course, important to remember that DCM is only used in the public or communal areas of a formal care setting, and observers do not intrude into private care settings such as bedrooms and bathrooms. And it is precisely in these latter areas that the majority of physical care tasks (such as toileting, dressing and undressing) are carried out. Even allowing for this fact, 2.5 per cent represents a very small amount of time, especially given that the clients in the in-patient unit were the most handicapped and dependent, and required the most practical support.

It was not surprising, then, that the day-hospital clients (who were relatively less handicapped and dependent) registered on average only 0.6 per cent of their time mapped at Green House as being in receipt of practical personal physical care (P). However, when the times mapped in the Green House minibus were included – both 'transport' to and from Green House and 'outings' – this percentage increased to 2.83 per cent. This was because considerable help and support were required to get people on and off the minibus, and arrange them comfortably and safely on board. For one client, Roy, on an outing, continual assistance was required since he was severely physically incapacitated by a stroke. So a staff nurse sat with her arm around him, holding in place the pillow which prevented him from banging his head against the window. The experience of watching the outside world in all its springtime glory, and of doing so in gentle and caring, physically supportive companionship was self-evidently a very positive one; his face was transfigured with joy, and his remarkable care score recorded the fact.

This was yet another example of the (unrecognised) positive experience which the Green House minibus provided. But with regard to the clients' views on dependence and particularly inter-dependence, one of the things which made the transport such a positive experience for clients was that problems could, and did, occur. The usual difficulties could be experienced loading wheel-chairs onto the tail-lift, and fitting people into the minibus in such a way that all disabilities were catered for. Additionally, the narrow lanes of Riverford and its surrounding villages provided more than ample scope for problems for the driver (usually the porter, whose excellent relationship with all the clients always made the journeys a happy experience).

However, on the porter's day off one of the day-hospital staff would drive instead. All the staff had been trained to do this and passed the necessary test. Nevertheless, they were much less familiar with the task. Turning the minibus around in a small lane could become a challenge for all its occupants – staff and clients alike. Clients' eyes and experience were then actually needed, as the travelling microcosm of cared – for and caregivers backed gingerly into gateways and nosed through narrow lanes. The collective sense of achievement after the successful outcome of such adventures was tangible, as all rediscovered in their present experience that, as Samuel had put it: 'We all rely on each other.'

The transport mappings highlighted some interesting inconsis-tencies with regard to clients' experience of physical dependency and of care. For while more handicapped clients in the relatively impover-ished social environment of the in-patient unit had far lower care scores and spent only 2.5 per cent of time receiving physical care, those less handicapped clients in the day-hospital received very much *less* physical care, but their care scores were far higher – due largely to the considerable amount of non-task-oriented interpersonal interaction (A). These care scores, however, were greatly increased during transport times, when the average percentage of time spent receiving practical physical care (P) also increased from 0.65 per cent to 2.83 per cent. Therefore, the practical physical care contributed to this increased good experience of care. And the occasions when clients themselves could also contribute to the overall welfare of *all* the occupants of the minibus (interdependence) were also observed precisely during these journeys. Physical care in response to practical needs, therefore, was only part of the overall story of clients' experience of dependence.

## Conclusion

The crucial factor which affected clients' experience of care in the Green House service was their level of handicap. Those who were still able to talk and retained social skills had a measurably different experience of care from those whose abilities had already been significantly eroded by organic degenerative brain disorder. This was the loss which most affected the quality of care delivered. It was the loss which, by implication, was most recognised by staff. For they distinguished between more and less communicatively able clients, both in their assessment of a client's awareness and also in the manner and style of care delivery. Even the language of the service discriminated between *clients* of the day-hospital and *patients* of the residential area. Since clients' experience of dependency was naturally related to their ability levels, this meant that those who were least able, and therefore most dependent, had the poorest perceived experience of care, as measured by indicators of well-being. And this could be seen to relate to increasingly withdrawn behaviour. 'For whosoever hath, to him shall be given, and he shall have more abundance: but whosoever hath not, from him shall be taken away even that he hath.' (Matthew 13:12).

# CHAPTER 6

# What other people said

*What were the perspectives of the other people involved with the Green House service? In particular, what did they have to say in relation to the themes which emerged from the interviews with clients? And can anyone but the client be 'the client's voice'?*

## Introduction

At the beginning of this book we looked at the two pictures of 'The Regents and the Regentesses of the Old Mens Almshouse' by Frans Hals. All we know of them is from Hals' portraits, that is, from his perspective. If, however, we had been able to talk to them ourselves about how they saw the old men and their almshouse, what might they have said? I do not want to suggest that those who managed and ran Green House necessarily resembled Hals' sitters in any way other than their responsibility for running a service for dependent elderly people. My point is that while Hals' point of view has been preserved, his sitters' has not. And in evaluating Green House I wanted to build as rounded, multi-dimensional picture of the service as possible. So although I privileged the perspective of the service users – the clients – I was also keen to hear what the other people involved had to say. In particular, when I looked at these interview records subsequently, I wanted to explore the ways and degrees to which the four over-arching themes which arose from the clients' interviews were reflected or recognised in those of the staff, the managers and the family carers.

So I interviewed as many of them as possible, individually and in depth. These interviews tended to take on average about two hours – some slightly less, some considerably more. I used a schedule or topic guide which I adapted slightly for each group. This was more to do with shifting the emphasis towards those areas which one could reasonably expect each group to know more about, although everyone was given the opportunity to discuss all the topics. I used open-ended questions. In my own mind I used the analogy of an estate agent showing someone round a house. I took my respondent into the house, and then opened the door into each room, inviting him or her to comment on the room – its size and shape and colour, etc. I tried not to 'lead' my respondents, but to give them space and encouragement to say what they really thought and felt. Unlike the interviews with clients, however, I did not make recordings but used my secretarial skills to take down what was said verbatim as far as possible. At the end of the interview I read my notes back so that people could have the opportunity to change, add or delete anything. I felt it was important that the interview record should accurately reflect both our understandings of what had been said.

When all the interviews were completed, I subjected the full record for each group to content analysis, looking both for what was actually said, for what was implied, and for significant ommissions. From this process there emerged a profile of responses from each group. As you would expect, for some topics I found general agreement, for others a limited variety of responses, and for others certain well-defined response clusters accompanied by a few 'outliers'. Taking all these topic profiles together, a characteristic group profile for each of the groups finally emerged.

## The interviews
*Staff*

I interviewed 29 staff of Green House, drawn from all disciplines with 'hands-on' client contact: nurses (qualified and unqualified), occupational therapists (qualified and unqualified), doctors, psychologists, domestic and portering staff. Only two people refused to be interviewed. Initially I faced staff hostility to my proposal to talk to the clients themselves. This idea was greeted with some suspicion by clinical staff, manifested in a 'coolness' of manner and a patronising attitude. Many of them explicitly voiced their disbelief in the possibility of my being able to interview or gain any feedback from clients. If they, with qualifications and experience, were unable to do this, how could I, as a mere amateur, hope to do so? It was also a problem, as well as an advantage, that I already knew, and was known by, most of the staff I interviewed. Although I benefited from existing and previous working relationships and familiarity, there was a certain difficulty in being accepted by people in the unaccustomed role of researcher. However, the situation altered dramatically when the nursing staff entered into a formal dispute with management over, among other things, staffing levels. All the unions were involved, and overnight the atmosphere at Green House changed. To my surprise, on my next visit there I was greeted with open arms and welcomed into the day hospital with warmth and appreciation. The staff welcomed the opportunity to 'off-load' onto a neutral observer, particularly in the privacy and confidentiality of the interview situation. Indeed, one senior nurse subsequently suggested that I would be welcome to interview all her staff on a regular basis, and that this could replace supervision, since they were noticeably more cheerful and enthusiastic on their return to work!

*Managers*

In all, I interviewed 17 managers connected with the setting up and running of Green House. No one refused. They were inevitably a disparate group, consisting of general managers of very different levels, financial administrators, technical services managers, support services managers, clinical line managers. The differences between them in terms of experience, expertise, seniority and educational background were considerable. Nevertheless, from their interviews it was clear that they shared understandings and viewpoints to a remarkable degree. Everyone took considerable trouble really to think about the issues put to them, and to give thoughtful answers. However, psychotic amnesia had to be a suspected diagnosis in a few cases! For Green House was in many ways a 'hot potato' at the time (as we have seen in Chapter Three), which aroused deep emotions in many of those concerned. The lack of agreement over the design of the building, which reflected the stop–start nature of its history, was one example. Another was the delay in finishing the building, which had resulted in very frail elderly clients having to make an interim move with a concomitant 50 per cent mortality rate. Where feelings of regret and remorse were explicitly and movingly expressed by some, others 'forgot the details', or passed over the incidents with extreme brevity, concentrating on less inflamatory topics at great length.

*Carers*

Strong feelings associated with difficult and painful memories were naturally very much a characteristic of my interviews with carers. Twenty carers of both day-hospital and in-patient unit clients agreed to be interviewed; three refused. I accepted Green House's own definition of 'the carer' – that is, the relative or contact that the primary nurse identified. In most cases this was a spouse, son, daughter or daughter-in-law of the client. In one unusual instance, however, it was the manager of the residential home where the client lived. They were all struggling in varying degrees with very considerable emotional, physical and economic stresses. And those who were not quite so encumbered might well be coping with feelings of guilt and resentment. Many carers were themselves elderly, and by virtue of their caring role they did not have a great deal of spare time to devote to being interviewed. This being the case I was very conscious of asking them to devote at least two hours, plus considerable intellectual and emotional effort, to a project which would not necessarily have any effect on their situation or that of their relative. And they were also vulnerable because of their dependence on the Green House service, so I felt it was important that they should feel no compulsion to cooperate with the evaluation. Certainly they might feel concerned about the confidentiality of the process, and I would inevitably be entering family situations, the dynamics of which would be partially or even largely unknown. They were watching loved ones apparently deteriorate before their eyes, truly able to understand neither what was happening nor why it should happen to them. Not surprisingly these interviews were emotionally taxing both for them and for me. When at the end I read back my notes to them, I often felt wary of having to read back certain parts of the interview to someone who had been upset (sometimes in tears) at that point. Yet I discovered that listening to their words (and their feelings) repeated back in another's voice seemed to bring calmness, as they would nod and confirm that that was exactly how they felt. I always tried to steer our conversation back into happier and more prosaic waters before I left, and all my respondents in each group received a 'thank you' letter.

## About awareness

*Staff*

The staff group's views on their clients' awareness were particularly interesting, given the context of their views on *management's* awareness of themselves. They were unanimous in accusing management of not including them in decisions about their own work: 'Decisions are made without knowledge or consultation.' Or again: 'We are never told the outcome of discussions – I call it "cloak-and-dagger" management!' Staff were united in feeling ignored and unappreciated: 'We work hard and we're understaffed, and we don't get any thanks. And it's especially important when you're struggling.'

With regard to their clients' awareness, their views focused around two things: the shortcomings of the physical layout of the building, and clients' ability to communicate in words. With regard to the building, much concern was expressed about the lack of a separate entrance for the day-hospital, since this meant that day-hospital clients had to process through the in-patient lounge in order to gain access to their own part of the building. This was seen as evidence in bricks and mortar of a total disregard for clients' sensitivities: the architecture itself was a denial of client awareness. For who would expect their own living-room to double as an entrance corridor for complete strangers? Two-thirds of the staff were of the opinion that Green House should have been designed for the convenience of the clients first and foremost, and there was strong feeling therefore at the invasion of in-patient privacy which the layout of the building forced on them. And they also understood the distress caused especially to day-hospital clients by their awareness of 'the other side'. The staff respondents heartily disliked the glass partitions dividing the two halves of the building, which meant that both client groups could see through into the other part, and these were explicitly recognised as a cause of client distress. Another perceived insult to client sensitivity was the fact that many clients had to share bedrooms, since there were only a few single occupancy rooms.

Many of the staff described a two-tier system of care, where the whole question of client awareness was used to explain the differences in practice between day-hospital and in-patient unit. Day-hospital clients were given more choices 'because they were more aware'. And their awareness was recognised – or not – by their ability to speak up: 'it depends which client goes to the toilet whether the door is shut or not. It's not right. If they can't speak for themselves they are not treated as individuals.'

However, many staff responses to a variety of topics indicated that they saw themselves, as it were, as extensions of the clients' own awareness. For instance, they were concerned to safeguard clients' personal dignity for them: 'Dignity is observed by maintaining courtesy, and the private needs of people.' They understood their role as supporting clients' dignity and privacy for them – being aware of these things on their behalf – when they could not do so for themselves. Many also indicated their wish to understand their clients better:

> We try to find out their background and provide activities to suit. It is very difficult if you don't have enough information.

Particularly those who can't communicate very well. We
need to know their interest and beliefs, and we don't
necessarily have enough information on them in the notes.

In part owing to this desire for better information, staff stressed the
importance of their relationship with family carers – 'we are their
lifeline' – painting a picture of a symbiotic relationship. They were
very sensitive to carers' emotional difficulties 'because the client is not
the person they knew'. For several of the staff the carers were the
people for whom they were really providing the service. More
mainstream was the view that carers provided crucial information
about individual clients, which the clients could no longer communicate for themselves. So staff saw carers as representing the client's
voice in its seeming absence, and themselves as the guardians of their
dignity in the seeming absence of their own awareness.

### Managers

Most of the managers I interviewed expressed commitment to a
'client-centred' and 'needs-based' approach to service provision and
care delivery, and believed the facilities should be designed primarily
for the convenience of clients. The possibility of client awareness
lurked as a lingering doubt – 'a small worry' – around much of what
was said. 'These patients may be aware of more than we think' said
one person. Yet managers showed only a very partial understanding
of clients' needs as they (the clients) themselves had expressed them.
In particular, far from realising the assault on clients' sensibilities
which the juxtaposition of day-hospital and in-patient unit caused,
most managers were in favour of such an 'integrated' facility. They
produced good management reasons – but these concerned the staff
rather than the clients:

It's organisationally simpler: one manager in control. It
avoids duplication. The consequences of working on one site
are a better service, and the support services are easier. A
bigger staff group has spin-offs: supporting each other,
stimulating good practice, training and morale.

However, they did also believe that 'it's a good idea from the client point of view, because day-hospital clients may eventually come in for respite care'. This was the often-voiced, fond fantasy that somehow increasing short-term memory loss would not prevent clients of the service from getting used to Green House. So when their memory became so impaired that they could no longer function safely even in their own home, they would nevertheless find Green House reassuringly familiar – thus achieving a seamless transition along the downward path mapped out for them. In other words, the clients of this narrative were a figment of managerial (and sometimes clinical) imagination. However, the 'small worry' surfaced again for a minority (one in five) who expressed doubts about integrated units, precisely on the grounds of a mutually unacceptable mix:

> Respite and continuing care should be separate. Continuing care means that it is a person's home. It should be separate within the unit, because it is like imposing holiday-makers on someone's home.

Several managers showed imaginative sensitivity to clients' own awareness of their confusion, and of the 'very demeaning' feeling of being dependent. And most managers were extremely wary of new integrated units attracting stigma in the community, thereby re-creating 'the institution'. And when it came to discussing choice, dignity and privacy they showed remarkable sensitivity and insight, explicitly identifying themselves with these issues:

> We maintain their dignity for all our sakes. If we don't care for theirs, we aren't caring for our own. Dementia is a loss of what seems to make us human ... Through valuing them, we value one another.

They also admitted that concern for carers' sensitivities was a prime motivation: 'it's the carers – they notice!' Indeed, carer awareness was cited by some as a salutory informal audit mechanism. But there was no recognition of clients' identity-supporting needs, nor that they might be dealing with the prospect of their own approaching death. Yet these are issues which have strong implications for service planning, with resource implications in terms of increased establishment, training and psychology service support. For other terminally ill people the hospice movement has long since demonstrated the value of recognising clients' psychotherapeutic and spiritual needs as they consciously approach the end of their life. It was here that the difference came out most clearly between a service that is motivated by a general awareness of 'good' humane values and of responsibility to the community in general and relatives in particular, and one that is motivated by a clear acceptance of client awareness. Caring for someone because *not* to do so would undermine one's own value-system and self-perception differs from doing so because one is in no doubt that their feelings and needs are the same as one's own.

### Carers

And the carers, of whose sensitivities both staff and managers were so conscious, how did they perceive their relatives' awareness? Despite forming a very diverse group of people, each of whom provided some highly individual perspectives and insights, interestingly, the single common area for all the carers focused around the issue of awareness and the parallel one of recognition. Whereas staff had used verbal communication skills as their measure of awareness, for relatives it seemed to be about recognition. This was either about the client's inability to recognise them: 'She often doesn't recognise me', 'She shows little interest – people don't register with her'; 'a cabbage, who can't recognise the people who come to see you!' Or it was about the carer's inability to recognise the client: 'They're so different to how they were – very moody, very difficult'; 'Not the person you used to know!' and even 'She's a complete zombie. Can't do anything – talk, walk, feed herself, go to the toilet, dress herself. She's like a baby with no animation – brain-dead!' It was here, in this nexus of mutual lack of recognition between those who had previously been (in most cases) the closest of relatives, that the most poignant picture of dementia emerged: the dislocation of relationship.

Many carers chose to frame things in terms of culturally prevalent concepts such as brain death: 'It's as if his brain has worn out'; 'It's [client's name] with his brain nearly gone – but he's still there.' As with the managers' 'small worry', permeating many of my interviews with carers was the hope of a client's continuing awareness – their presence: 'She's unable to express what she feels. But I'm sure the words are inside her but she can't get them out. It must be frustrating.' 'It's a very, very sad thing. So traumatic for them. They can't concentrate. They're in another world of their own. It must be terrible for them – because they do come to themselves sometimes and then realise what's happening. He said "I've been ill, haven't I?"' Perhaps this is why a third of the carers I spoke to said they would wish to be killed if they were to develop dementia: 'Shoot me!' Yet carers identified their relatives' needs as 'love', 'company', 'patience, kindness and understanding'; 'They need to feel as much a part of the world as they can.'

Consequently, carers brought this question-mark about their relative's awareness to bear upon both their opinion regarding the building, and the manner of care delivery which they witnesssed. For instance, they shared staff dissatisfaction with the physical layout of the building: 'I would prefer the respite care to be separate. It's better not to mix the respite people with continuing care.' 'I knew someone who was very distressed to see people wandering and spitting.' '"Am I really like these people?" That's what they think. The day-hospital and the in-patient side should be separate.' And they confirmed the DCM observations which showed a two-tier culture of care. One carer drew the comparison between where she worked as a volunteer and the in-patient unit where her husband was: 'Where I go to do the coffee in this residential home, they are treated differently to people who are senile, because they can answer back and won't accept what isn't right. A senile person has no say – so the staff treat them differently.' But the majority of carers were impressed with the standard of care they witnessed: 'They do the best they can with difficult patients.' 'The nurses are of a gentle and kind nature – it is the most saintly work to do – and it's people's feelings that come over.' There were definite concerns about gender-appropriate practices, showing that both carers' sensitivities and their view of clients' awareness were not always uppermost in care delivery: 'I'm not too happy about men handling my wife.'

## About the importance of other people

*Staff*

Staff were more conscious of the negative potential of the social environment for clients than its positive attributes: 'We don't all want to be together all the time – its a stress factor.' The fact that so many clients so greatly valued the congenial company of other people, and that this was extremely important to them for its own sake, did not appear to be consistently recognised by staff. They saw the value of relationship as far as carers were concerned, and their own role in supporting carer–client relationships, but as far as the significance of their relationships with clients was concerned, this was more often seen in an instrumental light; that is, for obtaining better information for the job. 'Stimulation' rather than relationship were the focus of concern for staff:

> The most able clients are in the day-hospital, and their care is intensive because we are trying to stimulate what they have, and give them more than they would get at home – something better than one-to-one care at home. The in-patients are the most handicapped and it requires a tremendous amount of effort and time to make their behaviours and handicaps as better as possible ... No one needs less than a lot of input.

There was a strong flavour of 'doing unto' rather than 'being with' in these interviews. The benefits of companionship per se seemed largely unrecognised.

A striking example of this was the way in which, as we have seen, staff respondents did not appreciate the hugely positive experience of personal care and attention which the daily journeys in the minibus afforded the day-hospital clients. Yet staff would say that their clients needed 'love and cuddles!' One person said, 'We are their contact with the outside world; what we give them is their world.' While this reflects a significant insight into the importance of their interpersonal contact with clients, nevertheless it was always framed in a unidirectional way. They saw themselves as the givers, and the clients as receivers. No one spoke of what the clients gave them.

Despite the great compassion with which staff spoke (often very movingly) about their clients' needs, implicitly there seemed to be a lack of acceptance of clients as people like themselves. And yet, coming in from the outside, as it were, when I read through all the staff responses I was very struck by what they said about the causes of their own distress in their work situation (particularly with regard to under-resourcing and the whole area of their relationship with management), their reactions to it, and the ways in which they needed to cope with it. Causes included: 'not being listened to'; 'not being able to air one's views'; 'the them-and-us situation'; 'not knowing what is going to happen'; 'frustrations at not being able to do what you set out to do'. And in their reactions also they described behaviours analogous to those observed in clients, such as withdrawal: 'I keep out of people's way!' or 'Bottling things up'; aggressive reactions: 'By getting bad-tempered!'; somatising: 'People get ill!'; and even escape: 'By leaving!' One respondent pointed out that 'Recognition [of stress] only comes here when something goes wrong!' (In the same way as I had observed that client behaviour was 'managed' reactively.) Similar also was the way some staff cited the importance of personal contact and support as ways of dealing with stress: 'By people talking to each other'; 'By sharing problems'; 'By laughing and joking about it – there's a lot of this about in order not to lose our tempers!' However, no one suggested they saw an analogy between their own experience of distress and that of their clients.

*Managers*

The importance of familiarity expressed by clients was recognised by many of the managers I interviewed. Indeed, it formed the basis of the justification for local units such as Green House. However, their overriding concern to avoid the evils of institutionalisation appeared in some way to constitute a barrier to a fuller understanding of clients' personal interaction needs which, as we have seen, went far beyond questions of unit size and service design. For the disruption caused by memory impairment meant that for clients the quality of each present moment was paramount, and this was surely why the importance of kind and familiar individual others, prepared and available for a communicative relationship, was the second most important feature of their interviews. Managers' focus on institutionalisation centred around the building design: 'I'm bitterly disappointed'; 'It looks like Sainsbury's'. Principally the question of individual bedrooms exercised them: 'People need their own identifiable personal space: non-invadable without invitation'; 'Everyone needs time alone.' While this is certainly true, it was also true that the clients I spoke to overwhelmingly longed for warm social contact. One person said: 'It is important to be kind', and several managers talked about their concern that staff were under-resourced and under-supported in their very challenging role: 'Any service should be staffed so that the needs of people can be met.' 'We must allow staff to practice so they don't feel they are jeopardising standards. Also, when they are tired they become demoralised … The staff are too knackered.'

While recognising staff as supporters and facilitators, the managers I spoke to did not express any great conviction about the overriding importance of personal interaction for clients. Nor did they show an understanding of their potential loneliness. Being in a facility in close proximity to former home and family was seen by them as sufficient guarantee against this, but the fact that ease of access did not of itself bring relatives in to visit regularly, and that clients could experience great isolation within the in-patient unit in particular, was not recognised. However, almost all these managers were in favour of small local units like Green House precisely because they supported people staying within their own homes and networks for longer, by providing day-hospital and respite facilities. This was very much interpreted as being about supporting relatives – 'They are the client's voice.'

*Carers*

Given their own painful insight into dementia as a dislocation of relationship, it is not surprising that carers showed far greater insight into clients' interpersonal contact needs than either staff or managers: 'There are a lot of lonely people', and 'They need to feel as much a part of the world as they can'. Carers were aware, as we have seen, of the negative aspects of social contact, in particular the problems of the juxtapostion of the day-hospital and in-patient unit, and the reaction of respite care clients to those more handicapped already receiving continuing care. However, much of what they had to say also related to wishes for greater interactional opportunities for the clients: 'Staff ought to know more about stimulating people – keeping alive what is there as long as possible. The way a person is looked after will affect the rate of deterioration.'

It was very much with their relatives' social contact needs in mind that they were happy to make suggestions as to how care at Green House could be improved. Overall, these suggestions clustered into five areas. First was the feeling many people expressed that clients should be able to go out and about in the world more than the little that they did: more walks, more exercise, more fresh air and sunshine, more normal social activities – they should be able to go out 'for a quiet tea somewhere – you'd have to warn the café in advance!' Second, carers wanted more of what they tended to refer to as 'intellectual stimulus'. Clearly the atrophy of brain functions which they saw as taking away from them the person they knew had to be slowed down as much as possible. Third, several of the carers were also very concerned about medication levels. They were worried about side-effects. But they also made the point that 'It makes it difficult to measure what is happening', and they felt that medication was being used as a way to manage behaviour, rather than finding solutions in relationship. The fourth suggestion referred to clients' 'need for spiritual comfort'. Several carers expressed this concern, and wished for clients to have the opportunity to attend church, or receive spiritual support in Green House. Finally, there was considerable clamour for clients to have access to counselling services: 'They need someone to talk to. The doctor doesn't have the time.' 'Perhaps a psy-chologist?' 'People need to talk about things and get it off their chest – and [the client relative] won't talk to me!' If the old relationships were proving difficult to sustain, there was at least a recognition by some people that supportive, communicative relationship was still a real need for clients.

## About loss

### Staff

One of the most notable features of the staff interviews was their movingly expressed insight into the importance for clients in the in-patient unit of the loss of their home. 'They are giving up their place in the world,' said one person. Others pointed out how particu-larly detrimental this loss was to those who were losing their memory: 'They are giving up the props to clarity,' and again: 'Home is so important because their past is their present identity – they live in the past.' Giving up home was variously described as giving up 'a lifetime's collection of everything!'; 'the ability to recognise things'; 'years of their life'; 'being able to shut your own front door'. Some people pointed out that people brought very few personal posses-sions in with them, even though this was supposed to be policy: 'They come in here and they have nothing!' All the staff identified closely with the meaning of 'home', and one echoed Norma, the client of the in-patient unit who supplied the title of this book, in speaking of home as the place to be yourself: 'You can't be yourself among others.'

Staff were genuinely concerned with the question of loss in some of its other forms. On the practical level they were aware of the problem of the loss of clothes and personal belongings which sometimes occurred in the in-patient unit – particularly with clients coming in for respite care. However, this they saw as a problem for carers (the carers agreed!), but not for clients. James, the sectioned client looking for his hat, and Mary, who so wanted her shoes back, had shown the importance and the deep meaning which clients attached to their personal things. Yet their disappearance was seen by staff as a matter for concern because it distressed relatives. On the other hand, their recognition of loss of faculties was concretely translated into a considerable preoccupation with preserving clients' dignity, privacy and choice. Staff very clearly saw their role as preventing loss of faculties leading to its most culturally unacceptable and disturbing manifestations. This was in tune with their view of themselves as somehow extensions of the clients: being aware *for* the clients, mitigating loss of faculties *on their behalf*.

But the most surprising gap in the staff interviews, given the amount of time they spent with clients, was the total absence of recognition of clients' sense of loss of their loved ones, and of the problems which their feelings of grief and bereavement posed for them in their confusion. Even when staff were asked to consider (in their view) areas of service dysfunction, there was absolutely no suggestion that counselling might be required. Yet given that memory problems meant that grief could constantly recur, clearly specialist insight and expertise were required. At that time the only recourse which staff seemed to feel they had was to a rather simplistic understanding of 'reality orientation,' as with the day-hospital client who was mourning both her father and her husband. This only produced further confusion for the client, as well as fear, as they were forced then to confront their own cognitive handicap and its implications.

### Managers

The managers I spoke to shared the staff's insight into the importance of the loss of home. A quarter of them described the function of Green House as being 'to reprovide home'. So they wanted it to be 'homely' and 'comfy' and 'a homely environment'. They believed that the day-hospital was the best way to keep people in their own homes. However, many of them also felt that the in-patient unit should be like 'a home for life' – something the clients who actually lived there clearly had not felt it to be. There were those who would have liked to provide care for everyone in their own homes, although they did not believe this to be possible.

Not all the managers involved with supplying services to Green House fully understood the client group it served. However, there was an appreciation of the fact that dementia meant a loss of 'the mental capabilities to remember who or where they are' as one person put it. Like the carers, they were very anxious that clients should be helped to retain their remaining abilities. But there was absolutely no mention by anyone of the fact that clients could be experiencing – and re-experiencing – the loss of loved ones. I think that it had not occurred to them that people so confused could be painfully cognisant of their bereavements, just as it had not occurred to people that clients had a sense of their own approaching death. However, the whole question of loss of things like choice, privacy and dignity was something which managers took very seriously indeed. Interestingly, clients in their interviews had made no explicit mention of this. This might have been because their experience of care was such that they were not aware of any loss of these things. But the negative aspects of social contact they referred to would suggest that loss of privacy at least was an issue for some clients. And similarly the theme of dependence would seem to indicate that loss of dignity was also an issue. As for loss of choice, it would seem that this was something that was important to other people – and not wrongly so – but that other things were much more important for the clients themselves.

*Carers*

In fact, it was the carers who most closely mirrored the clients' own expressions of loss, although even they seemed unaware of their bereavement needs. They agreed with staff and managers about the significance of the loss of home for clients. A third of them said that they would have preferred to have support provided at home, rather than have their relative go in for respite care. With regard to loss of faculties, there were some complaints that people had become even more handicapped after they came in to Green House: 'He was walking when he came in here. They put him in a chair and now he can't. But it would have been better for his brain and his digestion to have kept him walking.' They were in agreement with staff and managers about loss of dignity and privacy. They saw little point in questions of choice as a realistic option for people with cognitive impairments such as their relatives had. And as we have seen, clients themselves never mentioned it or intimated that this was of importance.

What differentiated carers from staff and managers were their focus (not unnaturally) on loss of relationship and loss of rights. The latter focused around the question, which was already arising at that time, of the provision of continuing care being inappropriate for the health service, although 'My mother worked hard, and dad paid in the stamps!' One very elderly carer, who was facing large private nursing home fees as a result of his wife's assessment at Green House, told the story of his neighbour of the same age, whose wife had had cancer. Her care had been assiduously provided by the health service over several years. Why, he asked, should he now be facing having to lose his home and much of his income because his own wife's condition was dementia and not cancer? He was overcome by the unfairness of the system which had added financial burdens to the terrible emotional loss and guilt he clearly felt at being no longer able to care for his wife himself at home: 'If I could get some help she needn't go into a nursing home. I'd do anything to have her home.' Indeed, the loss of which carers were most conscious was the broken relationship with their relatives. This was most painfully symbolised for them, as we have seen, when their loved one appeared no longer to know who they were.

## About dependence

*Staff*

What was staff's awareness of or sensitivity to the feelings that dependence can inherently engender in clients? One thing in which staff and managers agreed was their lively antipathy to 'institutionalism'. I came to think of it as the 'I' word, since it was always used as the worst insult ascribable. 'De-institutionalising the environment' figured prominently in staff criticisms of the design of

Green House, and the continuance of any institutional ambiance there was ascribed to faults in the building rather than care practice, although staff cuts were also blamed.

With regard to the parental analogy that was such a feature of clients' interviews, it appeared that such an understanding of the care relationship was implicit among the staff also. Some defined their role as 'carer' or 'interpreter'. Most used the words 'support', 'assist', 'preservation' and 'responsibility.' Over half described their own function in terms of 'looking after' and 'caring for'. As we have seen, there were references to 'love and cuddles'. Clients' needs were described as 'care', 'safety' and 'preservation from danger'. Several people emphasised that clients needed a 'homely', 'familiar', 'friendly' social environment. Added together, these descriptions of staff function and client need present a picture of nurture and responsibility within a warm and domestic framework, which certainly seems consonant with the parental analogy derived from the memory-stories of the clients' interviews.

Occasionally there were signs that some individuals recognised this picture and its concomitant dangers:

> Nurses try not to take everything away from them. They are asked if they want a drink, or to go to bed – yes or no. They are not forced. If they look tired they are still asked if they want to go to bed.

There were those who mentioned clients' need to keep their self-esteem, their confidence, their dignity and even 'to be understood'. These responses seemed to be reaching towards a different understanding of the caring role, which would be more focused on the emotional and psychological needs of clients with dementia. The practical expression of such a focus was touched on by staff commenting on the need to preserve privacy, dignity and choice. Here there were echos of Charles' and Samuel's concern for a more equal relationship. People spoke of 'not talking down to people' and 'not treating people in a flippant way and jollying them along (I wouldn't like that!)'. But this concern for the preservation of good manners in the care relationship was still not seen as being rooted in a more egalitarian concept of care, the 'give and take' that Charles had loved. Only one of the 29 staff I interviewed spoke of

> the unfortunate view of society that independence is so valued and dependence is so pitied. We need to recognise that we are all dependent in some way – and interdependent.

That was the one and only reference to interdependence by a member of staff, although there were many references to collaboration with other professionals, other agencies, and with carers. But no one considered including clients in the collaborative process, as case conferences, for instance, would be too 'daunting' or 'threatening' for them. 'We deal with the carers, and feed back the conclusions and discussions to the client as relevant.'

As with the themes of awareness and loss, there was an interesting implicit analogy with staff's own feelings about their dependence on management. For it seemed to staff that while compassion, respect for dignity, and consideration for their clients was required of them, they were not receiving these things from those on whom they were organisationally dependent. One person voiced what might be described as the 'trickle down' theory of care: 'Standards in care come down from the top!'

### Managers

Actually the view 'from the top' of client dependence was occasionally quite insightful. One manager described the clients of Green House as 'frightened people who can't trust themselves to look after themselves'. Despite the fact that almost all of them were very concerned to avoid institutionalisation, stigma and labelling (three of their pet bogeys, in fact!) this was the only manager to show this imaginative awareness that dependence can be inherently frightening – as we have seen that it was, for some of the clients at least – and that this is not necessarily lessened by the place in which care is delivered.

With regard to the parental analogy, how did managers see the Green House staff? It was most interesting that they seemed by implication to agree with it. Statements such as 'Staff know from

174 INCLUDING THE PERSON WITH DEMENTIA IN DESIGNING AND DELIVERING CARE

experience what is best for patients' have a certain ring of 'mother knows best'! Although some managers betrayed anxiety about staff training levels, for the most part they were happy to believe that staff were the best people to understand the clients and their needs, and to see that these were met.

Interdependence was nowhere an issue for the managers I spoke to. Collaboration, however, was. But the partners referred to did not include clients. This was not, therefore, the recognition of mutual worth implicit in some of the client interviews. Nor was it concerned with the fact that clients might feel a need to be needed. The care relationship was envisaged still as the traditional one-way street. People recognised the need for collaboration between agencies (health and social services) and framed their thoughts about community care and the question of local facilities often in these terms. And in bemoaning the design faults of Green House, blame was assigned to lack of coordination within the project team, and between the project team and the architect. When asked to comment on areas of service dysfunction, they highlighted lack of collaboration between professional groups, between agencies, between services, and between the health service and carers. But no mention was made by any manager of the potential dysfunctionality between the service and its clients.

In assigning to staff the awesome responsibility for assessing and meeting client needs, and for monitoring the results, managers gave no hint that they believed in the possibility of any counterbalancing information from the clients themselves. They effectively turned all the issues of care delivery – the 'how of care' – over to staff. It seemed that they were dependent on the staff too. The difference was that theirs was an elective dependence.

*Carers*

In listening to carers' views about clients' experience of dependence – and particularly in light of the parental analogy – it was significant that nearly half of the carers were daughters or sons of Green House clients. In other words, they had been themselves in a relationship of dependence with the person for whom they were now the designated 'carer', and who was now at least partially dependent on them. Similarly, we should note with regard to the issues of interdependence raised by some clients that a third of the carers interviewed were wives or husbands.

Since staff viewed carers as the voice of the client, it was perhaps more surprising that the carers I interviewed did not raise at all the issue of dependence and the feelings that it might engender in clients. Nor did they bring up the idea of interdependence and the desirability of a more egalitatarian approach to the care process. This would seem, therefore, to challenge the assumption that the voice of the client and the voice of the carer are one. But perhaps this absence of any discussion around issues of dependence was not so remarkable, given that the carers themselves could be seen as dependent on the Green House service. This they acknowledged with (often profound) gratitude. For example, when I asked about the benefits of Green House to them, 'rest', 'peace of mind', 'freedom', 're-assurance' and even 'the preservation of myself as an individual' were the sort of replies I received. One even went so far as to describe it as 'an indescribable Godsend!' The vast majority of carers were extremely positive about the way they were treated there, and even more so about the way the clients were treated.

However, beneath these generous (and genuine) accolades, closer inspection revealed a more complex picture. For, despite their ostensibly positive view of the staff and the service, the carers I spoke to also injected their concerns – which it appeared that their grateful-dependent role inhibited them from expressing directly through, as it were, the proper channels: the Green House complaints procedure. In fact, four out of five of them said they were quite unaware of this procedure. One person probably spoke for many with an honest admission of the 'bind' of dependence: 'Yes, I have complaints. But I don't want to upset [the client] because he is in their hands.' This underlying sense of their relative being, in a sense, a hostage, whose well-being could be compromised by their own overt criticism, would seem to be the maggot eating away inside the apple of collaboration with carers, so much prized by staff. And a quarter of these carers said that they had had communication problems with the service. One long-distance carer, for whom this would be particularly important, said of a case conference: 'Communication could be better. The meeting was organised at very short notice, and I didn't know what I was supposed to do – or what the purpose of the meeting was!'

In fact, carers presented at various junctures in their interviews quite a list of complaints. The most frequent concerned loss of clients' clothes (in the laundry) or personal possessions (such as glasses, or in one instance false teeth). Several had problems of access, and one in five had serious concerns about their relative's medication. There were complaints about inflexible respite care, and about the perceived inappropriateness of male staff performing personal physical care tasks for female clients. All these related to quite serious issues for both clients and carers, yet for the most part they had felt unable to voice them directly, and indeed had made no effort to discover the procedures for doing so effectively. While genuinely appreciative of the service, they were at the same time not secure enough in their own dependent relationship with it to lay claim to a right of criticism or suggestion. Unlike some of the clients I interviewed, however, they did not put in a plea for interdependence or collaboration.

Most interestingly of all, although three-quarters of carers said that they saw no disbenefits to themselves in the Green House service, and four out of five saw none to clients, nearly half of them, when asked about alternatives, opted for a nursing service in their own homes. Had such a system been operationalised, the domestic care setting would effectively have shifted the 'balance of power' in favour of carers, with nurses coming into carers' homes to work together with them. This would at least have provided a more effective collaborative ethos between staff and carers. Given the disempowered, grateful dependence of carers' relationship with staff, was this actually implicit in their suggestion?

Nowhere in the carers' interviews was there evidence of insight into the fear that the dependent situation could engender in clients, nor that clients themselves might wish for a more egalitarian care relationship. Carers' interpretation of clients' failure to recognise them as meaning that they were no longer 'aware' – that somehow the person was not 'there' anymore – no doubt prevented them from envisaging either of these things. Yet somewhere, for some carers, there must have been some suspicion of it. Nearly one-third, when asked: 'If it were you how would you wish to be cared for?' replied that they would wish to be killed. This seemed to intimate some apprehension of just how terrifying staying alive with dementia might be. However, a quarter of the carers I spoke to also answered this question by saying that they would wish to be cared for at Green House. And one respondent simply said that they would want ' someone who could understand my condition, and help me survive in it'.

In summary, then, carers appeared to show even less awareness of clients' feelings about dependence and interdependence than managers or staff. Their far greater personal pain in facing the suffering of (except in one case) a very close relative, their own distress (and no doubt guilt) at the limitations of their coping skills, and their extreme, grateful dependence on a service that went at least part of the way towards meeting their needs, all perhaps combined to prevent their perceiving the depths of clients' emotional world. Their pain was possibly so great that they could not even ask to be more involved in the planning and monitoring of care, although the list of their 'complaints' was significant.

## Conclusion

What are the lessons, then, to emerge from this overview of what other people involved with the Green House service had to say? I think, basically, there are two. First, that we need to understand those feelings and points of view with which we allow ourselves to identify. And second, that we need to be more alert to the limits of advocacy.

With regard to the first point, the most outstanding exemplar of this for me was the way in which all the staff I interviewed responded to the issues around the loss of one's own home. This, after all, is a situation with which just about everyone can imaginatively identify. Indeed, mortgages would probably not be repaid if we could not! So why was this sensitivity not translated into action? The DCM observations clearly showed that those clients who either had already lost their homes, or sensed they were about to do so (that is, the in-patient unit clients), did not experience a homely social environment full of warm and supportive personal interactions, whereas those who, for the most part, had not yet lost their own homes (the day-hospital clients) experienced precisely this.

The answer seems to lie in the different assessments of clients' ability to be aware of what was happening to them. This was 'measured' by staff in terms of their ability to communicate using language, and by carers in terms of their ability to recognise them. Those in the in-patient unit were by and large far less able in these respects; their awareness was consequently judged as being far less, and so the staff's imaginative identification with the plight of someone who has lost their own home was not extended to them. In other words, they were not considered sufficiently *sapiens*, as it were, to permit of being accorded the identification which we naturally feel for our fellow *homo*. This was all the more striking, given the analogous experiences of staff, managers and carers in relation to awareness, loss and dependence. It seemed that in their different ways each of these groups had first-hand experience of precisely the sort of issues with which the clients were preoccupied. Yet they did not perceive the analogy, nor, therefore, use it to help them understand their clients.

When it comes to understanding the limits of advocacy, I think these interviews provided a very telling argument for why we need to do our best to go straight to the source. If we wish to understand a certain point of view, then, in the final analysis, we can only do so by listening to the person concerned. Here we have seen why no one but the client can be 'the client's voice'. Managers tended to believe that staff knew about clients' needs and were their advocates; staff believed that family carers knew all about their client-relative, their wants and needs. Yet when we listen to individuals in all these groups we realise that everyone experiences 'dependence' in one shape or another, and that the perspective of each group is deeply affected by it. No-one can 'speak for' anyone else in a situation where each group has their own vital interest. In particular, it is also interesting to look at what we might call the 'elective dependence' of managers. Whereas staff and family carers had little choice in their dependence (staff on management for resources, carers on the staff and the service provided), managers tended to opt out of investigating the actual voice of the client. There seemed to be an assumption on their part that they did not possess the ability or skills to do so. My own lack of a clinical background did not prevent me from finding ways of doing this, and I believe this assumption needs to be challenged.

CHAPTER 7

# What can happen when we start to listen

*When those most closely involved with delivering care and planning services have the opportunity to observe and interpret the behaviour of older people with dementia, a measurable decrease in levels of ill-being can result.*

Perhaps the best part of the story of the Green House evaluation is that it had, if not a 'happy ending,' at least a positive and illuminating outcome. This outcome, in fact, grew not so much from the results of the evaluation as from one of its methods. It is to this outcome that we can now turn, for it provided a small indication of what might happen if people do indeed begin to listen – that is, when consciousness of the awareness and experience of clients themselves begins to be raised among those who work with and for them. For as a direct result of my using DCM as my observational tool, the health service Trust which ran Green House set up a project to investigate precisely this: what happens when staff and managers are given the opportunity and the skills to observe clients' actual experience of care?

As project manager I was responsible for training people and for implementing the use of DCM across five of the in-patient units for elderly clients with dementia. In all of this I was actively supported by Tom Kitwood, who came to conduct two large training courses, and made subsequent visits to monitor and encourage us all. His help with the analysis of the data towards the end of the project was invaluable.

The project also benefited from top-level support within the organisation, where the director of corporate development acted as project sponsor – or 'playing a hunch', as he preferred to put it! And the story of the Springton DCM project would not be complete without acknowledging the tireless and imaginative support given to it by so many staff who were *not* directly clinically involved, such as our management accountant and information analyst. We were allowed to use a disused ward for our training courses, and portering staff moved quantities of unwanted hospital furniture for us with no charge. Similarly the catering department kept us supplied with tea, coffee and biscuits – and never got round to invoicing for them, even when asked! The general level of support for what we were trying to do was palpable. It seemed as if everyone wanted the lives of our elderly clients with dementia to be better – and if this might be a way of achieving that, then they wanted to help. Indeed, part of the funding for the project was contributed from the end-of-year under-spend of a group of maintenance staff, who had liked what they saw happening on these wards and so thought we could use it better than they could.

But those primarily involved in the project were the majority of hands-on staff of all disciplines, many managers, and even two courageous family carers, all of whom were trained in DCM and given the opportunity to use it. The mappers included not only qualified and unqualified nurses but occupational therapists, psychologists, doctors, porters and domestic assistants. The project was funded in major part by money from the regional clinical audit. As it went on, it caused quite a buzz of excitement in the service and elsewhere. In fact, we were runners-up in the Hewlett-Packard 'Golden Helix' award for quality initiatives in health care in 1995.

I think the enthusiasm and the widespread interest which the project generated is worth noting. To my mind it showed the hunger that there is for just this sort of information. For those directly involved in delivering care are deeply curious about the experience of those they care for. They really want to know if what they are doing is 'hitting the spot'. After all, most people enter the caring professions because they want to make a real difference in alleviating human suffering. The apparent lack of feedback when nursing a very handi-capped elderly person with dementia can make the tasks of caring unrewarding and dispiriting. Learning to read the non-verbal com-munication of body language, and to explore *with* the patient those ways of supporting them which contribute to their well-being, can transform life for the caregiver as well as the client.

Entering into this world with both staff and clients was clearly not only rewarding and illuminating for managers, but often deeply personally moving also. For some of them it was about recapturing the motivation which had brought them into the health service; for others it was a whole new world. For all of them it provided a singular opportunity to understand not only the clients' experience but that of the staff – the daily challenges and stresses, and also the rewards of their work. The project furnished an acceptable context, and DCM a shared language, within which managers and staff could meet and share what they had seen and understood of how life was for people with dementia in their care. Venturing into the *terra incognita* of the experience of older people with dementia was emotionally chal-lenging, but also exciting, in that together we caught a glimpse of another world of caring towards which it is, in fact, possible to move. I think we only got to the entrance gate – but we looked in together and found the prospect inviting.

## How we put DCM to work

My own experience of DCM had been that it not only furnished valuable information with regard to clients' experience and their social and emotional needs, but also provoked in me, the observer, a radically new, enriched perspective of the care environment 'through the clients' eyes'. This was why I wanted to set up a pilot project to investigate the potential of DCM as a quality tool, using this con-sciousness-raising characteristic to effect a change in the practice of care delivery.

Five of the Trust's in-patient facilities were selected to take part in the pilot project, and one of these was the in-patient unit (but not, therefore, the day-hospital) at Green House. And so it was that new observational data about the in-patient facility at Green House became available two years on from my original evaluation. This time the observations were made by the staff of Green House, not just by me. From the charge nurse to the porter, all the staff of Green House who wanted to 'map' were trained in DCM and given the opportunity to use it. I recall only one person who did not want to do so. I should point out here that Tom and Kathy, who had designed and developed DCM, had subjected it to stringent reliability testing which established the inter-rater reliability of trained and experienced mappers as between .85 and .9. I should also add that since all those involved in the pilot project were trained personally by me (and initially accompanied by me during mapping) the inter-rater reliability of the results would appear to be trustworthy. There was, you might say, an equal 'contamination' of all mappers by the same party!

The idea behind the pilot project had been to make the use of this tool available to all staff with client contact: different clinical disciplines, qualified and unqualified staff, domestic and portering staff, and managers. Importantly, some very senior managers of the Trust (including the Chief Executive) learned and used this tool. So did the Quality Manager and the Chair of the local Health Commission ('the purchaser'). Those responsible for purchasing, planning, designing and running services (like Green House) for those with dementia needed to share the same window of insight as those whose delivery of care they purchased. Also, we all hoped that being in possession of a common language (DCM) in which to discuss service provision, and using a common understanding of clients' actual experience, would facilitate a shared vision for future planning. For DCM did, in fact, constitute a language; it was a structured way of looking at the care environment, reading behaviours within it, and recording these. Whereas clinical staff and managers each had their own professional languages, the learning and using of DCM served as a sort of 'esperanto.' Far from seeming intimidated, the staff appeared to welcome the opportunity which having a strategic-level manager 'mapping' on their ward afforded, both for demonstrating their skills and for meaningful discussions about client needs.

All those trained (staff and managers) tracked the experience of up to five individual clients for a period of between four and five hours – that is, most of a nursing shift. This involved a detailed observation of everything that happened (or did not happen!) to each client, minute-by-minute, and faithfully recording it according to the rules of the method. Towards the end of the shift the 'mapper' would spend about half-an-hour analysing the results, and then join the staff 'handover' session to feed back. In this way the information they were able to provide was fresh, relevant, and able to be used immediately in care planning.

## What changed

For each mapper it was a voyage into the world of the client, learning to see the environment as they saw it, watching the story of their lives in the care environment unfold moment by moment. It enabled them to perceive and understand, often for the first time, the reality of living with dementia from the clients' own perspective. For almost everyone this proved emotionally very challenging, as the comforting defence of being able to believe that clients were 'no longer aware' was steadily stripped away from them. That is to say, their own awareness of *client* awareness was radically altered.

By the end of the project, therefore, I was able to use this data, gathered from 'mapping' sessions at Green House over a period of four-and-a-half months, to investigate the effects (if any) of this raising of staff and management awareness of clients' experience. I did this by comparing it with the original DCM data from the in-patient facility. Three things emerged clearly from this comparison. In order to explain how we found them I shall need to refer in some technical detail to the concepts of the DCM method, as described in Chapter Two.

The first difference that emerged was an increase in the overall average care score from 'fair' to 'good', as shown in Graph 2. This meant that the average in-patient had moved from a 'fair' to a 'good' experience of care. Of course, this referred only to an average, and as two-and-a-half years had intervened since the original mapping, the composition of the client group had changed, although some clients from the original evaluation were still there. Consequently it was only meaningful to assess the clients of the in-patient unit as a single group, rather than the four categories I had originally used. Despite these limitations on the comparison, this nevertheless represented a real change in the average experience of clients in the in-patient area. It reflected a change, moreover, that was very noticeable on the

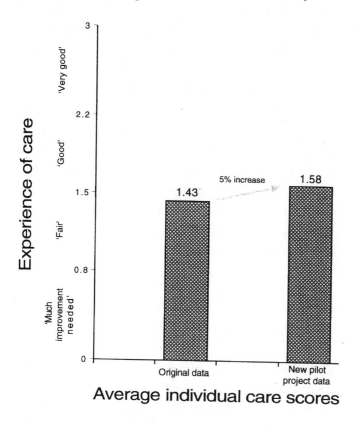

*Improvement in average individual care scores.*

ground. The in-patient lounge seemed a far more peaceful place than previously. The anxious wandering, rocking and calling out were much less apparent, and staff–client interactions seemed both more frequent and more focused. I particularly noticed the absence of 'over-the-client's-head' discussions between staff (hitherto the most frequent of the 'personal detractions' noted in the DCM observations). When a member of staff was with a client, it was *with* the client that they tended to have eye contact, and *to* the client that they addressed themselves.

The second difference was a dramatic reduction in the levels of 'slight ill-being' among clients. This emerged from a comparison of the different levels of well- and ill-being among clients recorded in the original evaluation and then in the project. DCM uses six levels of well- and ill-being to record in each five-minute time-frame. -5 is used to record severe ill-being; -3, moderate ill-being; -1, slight ill-being. +1 is used to record a 'maintenance' level, that is, where no ill-being is observed but nothing particularly positive either. +3 is for moderate well-being, usually but not necessarily involving personal interaction. +5 is for a 'highly therapeutic' experience. I built up 'Care Value Profiles', that is, added up every instance of each of the six well- and ill-being levels that had been recorded, to reveal the pattern of well- and ill-being. I then constructed an overall Care Value Profile from an aggregate of all the mapping sessions of the project, and did the same for all the original evaluation data. Then I compared them using chi-squared. This was the result:

|          | -5 | -3 | -1  | +1  | +3  | +5 |
|----------|-----|-----|-----|-----|-----|-----|
| Old data | 0% | 0% | 16% | 48% | 33% | 3% |
| New data | 0% | 0% | 8%  | 58% | 30% | 4% |

In order to demonstrate the changes more clearly I have given them here as percentages. However, chi-squared cannot be used on percentages, and was therefore applied to the original total figures for the incidences of each category (+1, +3, etc.). The two Care Value Profiles may also be demonstrated graphically (see Graph 3).

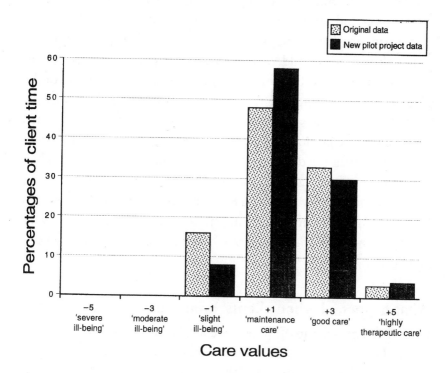

*A comparison of care value profiles from the original evaluation and the DCM project.*

The biggest difference was in levels of 'slight ill-being', which had been reduced by half. At the same time 'maintenance care' had increased by 10 per cent, and 'highly therapeutic care' by 1 per cent. These changes were statistically significant at the 0.01 level at 5 degrees of freedom. In other words, the likelihood of the change measured being due to the operation of chance factors was very slight indeed. This therefore represents a very significant measure of the changes in the clients' lived experience of care, achieved by increasing staff and management consciousness of clients' awareness.

The third change was in the balance of the activities recorded. On the one hand, eating and drinking had overtaken sitting just looking around as the most often recorded activity, and on the other, the amount of time when practical physical care was recorded increased almost threefold: from 2.5 per cent to 6.9 per cent. I discovered this by constructing 'Behaviour Category Code' profiles. Just as with the Care Value Profiles, I added up every instance of each of the different behaviours recorded, first for the original evaluation and then for the project. When I compared them, the first thing I noticed was the apparent *lack* of change. The three commonest behaviours recorded remained sitting just looking around (B), eating and drinking (F), and sleeping (N). But the difference was that eating and drinking (F) had taken over the first place from sitting just looking around (B). So we might say that instead of being a BFN environment, it had become an FBN one. And although practical physical care still occupied a very small percentage of the time, nevertheless it had increased very considerably.

## What happened when clients' awareness was recognised

What was the meaning of these three results? For those familiar with Green House the change in atmosphere was very perceptible. Anecdotal evidence suggested that 'on the ground' the difference in the 'feel' of the social environment appeared considerable, both to those who worked there and to those who visited. In other words, those of us, as it were, without dementia were very aware of a distinct change. Yet the changes seen when the observational data was analysed, though significant, were not as radical as I think we had all expected. True, the average care score had increased by a whole category, client 'slight ill-being' had been halved, and 'maintenance care' increased. Yet it could be said that the increase in average care score was only 0.15, and the episodes of 'good care' had actually slightly decreased. And the Behaviour Category Code profile was almost unaltered. At first sight this all seemed a little disappointing. I think we had all hoped to see our 'on the ground' experience confirmed in massive increases in 'highly therapeutic' levels of care, and concomitant dramatic leaps in care scores. But the DCM training and implementation was the only change introduced into Green

House during that time. There were no increased staffing levels, no additional training, no other extra resourcing of the unit of any kind.

Changing the culture of care is a long-term and a fragile process. And it still remains largely mysterious. I think that the picture which emerged from comparing the old and new DCM data represented a snapshot of the change process at its outset. It was rather like how a boat looks when it is just leaving the wharf – most of what is seen is the stern. The new image of the whole boat only becomes clear as it turns further out to sea. That is, what felt so striking a change in ambiance clearly did not, for example, translate instantly into a miraculous conversion of all negative Care Values into +3 ('good') and +5 ('highly therapeutic'). What the Green House comparative data shows is *how* the culture changes when it starts to do so, that is, the processes by which it shifts.

What seemed to have occurred was that those in contact with clients had become more aware of their emotional needs, and this had shown itself primarily in far greater overall attention to any signs of 'slight ill-being'. Whereas before the majority of clients in the in-patient unit had spent considerable time in this state, while the lucky few (those who were 'more aware') had benefited from 'good care,' now all clients spent far less time in it. Staff input would appear to have been redistributed from more concentrated interaction with an 'elite' of less handicapped clients, into ensuring that at least the *majority* of clients for the *majority* of the time experienced 'maintenance care.' In other words, learning to read clients' behaviour – effectively 'listening' to what their body language was communicating – had resulted in an acutely raised consciousness not just of the awareness of even the most handicapped, but particularly that this was often a *distressed* awareness. This had led to what we might think of as a 'utilitarian' response, whereby staff set out to ensure the greatest good of the greatest number. The difference of which everyone (without dementia) had been so aware was, I think, just this: the dramatic reduction in episodes of 'minor' distress.

If such a modest but highly significant change can 'feel' so different, the question raised has to be: how would an even greater change in DCM results translate in lived experience? Behind this question is another. If increasing staff and managers' awareness of their clients' experience can achieve this result using existing resources, what resources would it take to increase the +3 ('good care') scores and enrich the behaviour profile – that is, for clients to experience many more 'good' interpersonal interactions, and for their time to be spent doing other things than eating, looking around and sleeping? In other words, if the quality of clients' experience is to be taken seriously, what are the resource implications in service planning?

## What happened to clients' experience of social contact

Since only the in-patient unit was part of the DCM project, it was not possible to investigate any changes that might have occurred in the (more sociable) day-hospital, although new working practices meant that staff now worked more commonly in both areas, and so those trained in DCM were also working in the day-hospital. However, we have seen that within the in-patient unit clients' average care score had risen from 'fair' to 'good'. But did this entail an increase in the experience of friendly companionship? Were they less lonely?

Despite the dramatic reduction in 'slight ill-being' and the increase in 'maintenance care', no such positive change was shown in 'good care', which had, in fact, slightly decreased. This +3 Care Value usually denotes the greater quality of interpersonal interaction within a given context. For example, personal practical physical care (P) could have a Care Value of +3 if there was 'interactive assistance, conversation, etc.' (Kitwood and Bredin 1994), and eating and drinking (F) could have a Care Value of +3 if there were 'empowering assistance, moderate sociability, or obvious enjoyment' (Kitwood and Bredin 1994). How to explain, then, that increasing awareness of clients' experience (which in the in-patient unit was so often lonely) had not resulted in increased interactivity? I discussed this a great deal both with the staff concerned and with Tom. Given the absence of any other input (either more staff or more training), we felt that this should be attributed to the increase in staff awareness of client ill-being and the corresponding spreading of their time and effort more widely across the client group.

The high percentage of clients who were very physically frail or handicapped in addition to being confused was a significant feature of the in-patient facility. (The day-hospital clients, for instance, were far less physically dependent.) At one time during the project as many as two-thirds of the in-patient clients were extremely physically dependent. Consequently a very high proportion of staff time was taken up in ensuring that all the basic physical needs of each of these individual clients were met. As well as the significant increase in episodes of practical physical care, I noticed both the high degree of sensitivity and motivation which the use of DCM had induced.

Tom and I looked at the data long and hard, and formed the hypothesis that the staff seemed to be approaching the ceiling of what they could achieve in terms of both staffing levels and present interactional skills. It should immediately be said that the latter were in many cases very high indeed. Both qualified and unqualified staff demonstrated remarkable sensitivity, imagination and ingenuity in dealing with the most physically and cognitively frail clients imaginable. Getting through the physical workload while adding their new insights to their existing skills stretched existing staff resources close to their limit. The fact that they were so eager to continue with the project despite this was a great tribute not only to their professionalism, but to their humanity. Nevertheless, at the completion of the project, this was the extent of the change that had been possible – using existing resources, both in terms of staff numbers and present known interactional skills.

The change seen in the overall group Behaviour Category Code profile seemed to support our hypothesis, and also suggested an explanation. As we have seen, in the old data the most recorded activity for the in-patient area had been sitting just looking around (B), and over the life of the project it was overtaken by eating and drinking (F). This was an interactional activity, particularly in the in-patient area where so many of the clients required total assistance for both eating and drinking. Food would seem to be the care medium of choice in this sort of environment. That is, it was a visible means of expressing concern for well-being, and immediately rewarding, in that the results of care could be measured, so to speak, by the decreased amount of food left on the plate. We have seen in Chapter Five how, when a mapping period did not include a mealtime, clients' Individual Care Scores plummeted. In increasing the amount of client time spent in eating and drinking (F), then, staff motivation to increase clients' well-being took the (understandable) form of enhancing an activity which was already a strong point for them.

Walking about (K) and sleep (N) were the fourth and fifth most common codes respectively. It should be said that, over all the five in-patient wards taking part in the project, the group profile showed invariably a 'BFKN environment' (the order is alphabetic.) So Green House was not in any way unusual in this. This in itself, however, showed clearly the impoverished nature of the social environment in these in-patient wards for people with dementia. Green House was fortunate in having the part-time services of a qualified occupational therapist in the in-patient area as well as the day-hospital. This was not true of all the other wards. The message generated by this absence of occupational therapy for staff seemed to be that such areas represented 'the end of the line'. Nothing more could be done for these clients except to provide humane custodial care by meeting their basic physical needs. There seemed to be a meaningful symbolism in the fact that practical personal physical care (P) was the fifth commonest code recorded, and the one which had tripled during the lifetime of the project.

It was as if physical assistance, especially with eating and drinking, was still where staff concentrated their efforts – as in the traditional nursing models where clients' physical needs are what is assessed. But there was no great increase in episodes of personal interaction per se. Companionship for its own sake, and not simply because it was necessary within the context of the delivery of physical care, could still not be high on the agenda. The personnel and skill resources were insufficient.

Staff and carer respondents' concern for 'stimulation' had to be interpreted within this context – as a demand not just for more staff but for a greater variety of skills. Indeed, some of the carers' suggestions clearly showed this; for example, the need for counselling skills to be available for the clients of Green House. Another piece of supporting evidence came from a way of processing the DCM data which was called the 'Dementia Care Quotient' (DCQ). This was a calculation which incorporated the staff–client ratio with the average (or 'group') care score, so that higher staffing levels are effectively penalised, and lower ones rewarded. In other words, if a high average care score was recorded, the effect of a low staff–client ratio would be to moderate it by effectively saying 'If you only had so few staff, then this level of care represents quite an achievement.' And, of course, vice versa. This particular calculation has now been replaced in the DCM method. But at this time we were still using it, and my experience was that the DCQ gave the feedback from mapping increased credibility in the eyes of the staff concerned. It provided a realistic frame (a resource context), as it were, within which client care could be fairly evaluated. It accepted that care was the art of the possible. However, a comparison of the average DCQ for the original evaluation and then for the project at Green House showed only a relatively small increase (from 61 to 69). Given the significant changes in care scores and Care Value Profiles, the modesty of this result would seem to indicate that, with the best will in the world, staff had reached the ceiling of their interactional skills.

## What recognition was there of clients' experience of loss?

With regard to clients' expressed feelings of loss, did these changes have anything to say about whether or not these feelings were being acknowledged with increased insight or not? Certainly the fact that clients now spent half as much time in states of 'slight ill-being' would seem to indicate that staff were becoming more alert and sensitive to their depression and distress. The fact that −3 ('moderate ill-being') or −5 ('severe ill-being') had in any case been a rarity in the Green House DCM recordings is a tribute to the staff's already having been sensitive to higher levels of distress. The halving of the 'slight ill-being' scores, therefore, shows that their use of DCM had secured an insight into those (often extended) periods of sadness, melancholy, apathy and withdrawal which had originally constituted nearly a fifth of the in-patient clients' experience of 'care'. Within existing staffing and skill resources, a very creditable attempt had been made to alleviate these states. However, we have seen that this appeared to have been achieved somewhat at the expense of the 'good' (+3) experiences of the few. Nevertheless it represented an overall betterment of the client experience of care, and the fact that no one was left unattended, or at least marginally unconsoled, for very long.

Clients displaying sadness or the distress of grief, therefore, were now twice as likely to receive some personal attention. The fact that, as we have seen, sitting just looking around had been overtaken by eating and drinking, we interpreted as showing that staff fell back on those skills and interventions which their experience had shown them to be positive for clients, and which I had observed also provided positive reinforcement for themselves. The giving of nourishment was seen to be the most satisfying medium of care delivery for many staff members, and one in which their relationship with clients seemed clearest to them. Social interaction (A), however, remained as only the sixth most frequently recorded behaviour – still taking up only 6 per cent of in-patient clients' time. Although it would clearly be possible for counselling to take place while walking around (in which case it would be recorded as K) or within the context of other activities or physical care delivery, nevertheless it would be likely that the number of 'A' codings would increase significantly if a serious counselling programme to address clients' bereavement problems had, in fact, been attempted. This, however, was not the case. At no time did I hear of any such intention on the part of staff, or indeed that such specialist skills training had been identified as a training need.

In summary, therefore, while staff had become more aware of clients' sadness and apathetic states, and had begun to address them so that they were far less likely to be left alone in their distress, the full recognition of clients' emotional and psychological suffering had yet to dawn over Green House. No doubt the background awareness of insufficient staff with such specialist bereavement counselling skills for helping people with memory problems impeded this recognition.

## What was the effect on clients' experience of dependence?

The project data painted a picture of the care environment at a point of change. While a lot of ground had been covered towards the eradication of ill-being, the environment was not yet characterised by consistently positive interactions geared to support the personhood and well-being of individual clients. Tom's own yardstick for this 'new culture of dementia care' (Kitwood and Benson 1995) was that we would find that the 'good' (+3) Care Values were recorded more frequently than any others. There were one or two days during the overall project when we did, in fact, map such a culture. And we did not need to wait till the end of the session and count up our '+3s' to know it! The new culture is a very palpable thing, all too rarely experienced by any of us. The DCM project data for Green House still showed that +1 was the most frequently recorded Care Value.

How did this relate to clients' experience of dependence? The inference here can necessarily only be tenuous. However, it would appear to indicate that while the more obvious anxiety states of clients were definitely being addressed, their overall well-being was not at a level where their more subtle and profound concerns, such as the fear and sense of stigma engendered by awareness of their dependent status, were being answered.

However, we have seen that in two particular areas positive changes with regard to client dependency were recorded. These were the increase in recorded episodes of eating and drinking and practical personal physical care. We interpreted this as the result of the staff's recognition of the importance and significance for clients of personal interaction. Naturally, the first fruit of this recognition was concentration on those parts of the care process in which, as nurses, they felt most confident of their skills, that is, the giving of nourishment and of practical physical care, so that in the domain of practical dependence staff had very considerably upgraded their practice. Recognising the invaluable support which their presence and interactive skills represented in terms of clients' well-being, they had concentrated their efforts on those areas where they were most confident of achieving a positive change. Here again the data suggests a snapshot of the process of change at its outset. Everyone tends to begin by using the skills they already possess.

One other small but hopeful change that emerged from the comparison of Care Value Profiles has a possible bearing on clients' experience of dependence. According to the DCM method, 'highly therapeutic care' (+5) can sometimes refer to instances of one client's helpfulness to another. For example, I remember an occasion during the project when I was mapping with one of the staff, during which we witnessed the following scene. Two elderly men were sitting near one another – one of them was Joe, who was among the most handicapped clients there. He never spoke, and seemed unable to move by himself or feed himself. He began a fit of coughing, and continued coughing. His companion, Jerry, began by lifting his head, and then by asking 'Are you all right, mate?' As the coughing continued he then lent over to tap his afflicted companion on the back – as one does. And then he decided that further help was required, so he began to call out 'Nurse!' He was immediately answered, and Joe was helped to drink a little water. The coughing ceased. The nurse thanked Jerry. All three men sat companionably together for a while, and Jerry seemed well satisfied. His body language was very relaxed, and he was gently smiling. We, the mappers, coded his behaviour 'L+5.' For he had been involved in a crucial task: this was 'work' or 'labour' (L).

After all, if a nurse had assisted a client, that would be 'work'. Why was it not 'work' when a fellow client did it? This was certainly an example of interdependence of a sort. However, when we looked at the comparison of Care Value Profiles, we found only a 1% increase in such +5 moments (from 3% to 4%). While this was statistically significant, it was hardly an indicator that Green House had been transformed into an environment where care was 'a two-way street' (Barnett 1997). Nevertheless, it was a very slight movement towards this, in that the culture of care in the environment had allowed this encouraging episode to occur. For the nursing response had been entirely appropriate to what the client who called for help for his neighbour had wanted: help had been immediate, effective, and collegial.

Taken together, these changes indicated that in terms of practical physical dependence, clients' needs were beginning to be both recognised and addressed. But the more profound underlying emotional needs which confusion and helplessness can engender, particularly when the legacy of previous life experiences of dependence are taken into account, would require far more radical personal and organisational change.

## Conclusion

Looking at what happened at Green House when people began to listen to the clients' experience of care brings up several points. The first, and overwhelmingly positive, thing is the increased sensitivity to 'slight' ill-being, which led to such a dramatic reduction in it. For those of us who either worked there or who visited Green House for whatever reason, this halving of instances of slight ill-being brought about a very noticeable change in the whole atmosphere. Just eliminating the anxious wandering, rocking, calling out, and disconsolate, slumped withdrawal from the world had a wonderful effect on the whole environment. One can only hope that this change felt even better for the clients themselves. Certainly, the change in the overall environment should make the individual's experience more likely to be positive, since, as we have seen, this reduction in ill-being levels also translated into improved average Individual Care Scores. It also translated into a more equitable distribution of staff input, so that the more able clients perhaps received less input, but the less able recieved more. This has implications for resourcing. The Green House experience shows the limits of the attainable without increased input, in terms of both the staff–client ratio and of increasing skills. The staff operationalised their new insight and understanding of their clients' needs by focusing on their own tried and trusted skills and abilities, namely, assisting clients with eating and drinking and with personal physical care tasks. In order to move beyond this and be able to provide therapeutic companionship and special counselling, particularly for bereavement, further skills training was required. There is a very considerable difference between the skills needed to conduct the tasks of physical care with sensitivity and interactivity, and the skills needed to 'just be' for extended periods of time with someone with whom we may not be able to hold a conversation. And companionship is also, in part, about the gracious art of receiving: that is, of finding reciprocity in the relationship.

# CHAPTER 8

# The costs of care

*Looking at the emotional and psychological costs of care is more likely to show us how to improve dementia care services than a narrow focus on finances. Our time, our natural intuitive abilities and our imagination need to be invested in a new cooperative model of care. We need to be good companions.*

New insights and ideas do not walk around on their own; they come to us clothed in people. The search for social progress, service improvement, or even personal and professional growth necessarily involves encounters with new, and often unsettling, voices. If we are not open to other-ness, then we condemn ourselves to stale and circular thinking. This is as true in the field of dementia care as it is in any other.

Encounter with other-ness is what this book has described: older people's encounter with the prospects which increasing memory loss and cognitive impairment present, and their encounter, too, with society's response to their decreasing ability to remain 'homo *sapiens*'. It has also looked at the encounter of those relatives, care staff and managers involved in supporting them, with the problems and challenges which this handicap presents for *them* – for they too are people who cannot run away from the problem. And finally we have looked at the beginnings of a new encounter: that of those most closely involved with caring, as they step over the threshold into the world of those for whom they care. In doing so they also take their place in history: the long, slow, but persistent imperative for social inclusion, for discovering relationship, meaning and hope in the encounter with other-ness. For the other has always been knocking on the door, and pushing its point-of-view through the letter-box when the door remained closed. Some of these 'leaflets' have been more powerful than others.

For instance, we began by looking at two insightful and disturbing representations of 'care' in the seventeenth century. Frans Hals was an artist of great skill, and so able to portray those who administered alms to him in such a way that we can see as he saw, and feel what he felt. Consequently one frail and destitute old man's experience of care in a particular institution a very long time ago was etched on the consciousness of posterity. We look at his subjects and ask: 'How *can* they have been so distant, so cold?' If we had been there (we think) we would not have been so condescending. After all, what a privilege to meet (and be painted by) such a great artist! We have, of course, judged the man by his ability. We look at his work and marvel that the world of his time could leave a genius destitute. I wonder if, centuries from now (let us hope it will be sooner than that!), people will marvel that human beings could leave *any* of their number (genius or otherwise) so unincluded, so unrecognised in their common humanity, as we still leave people with dementia.

As we stand at the beginning of the twenty-first century, what do the clients of Green House have to say about *us*? In particular, what does the Green House experience have to say about why we should listen to people with dementia? I think it gives us three things to think about. It opens up both the question of awareness in older people with dementia and those who support them, and that of the therapeutic relationship and the dependent role. Both of these have resource implications in terms of personnel and skills. It also paints a picture of the costs of our present system of 'care'.

## Sharing our worlds

First, and above all, we see that elderly people with dementia in our care services do actually have a point of view: they are *aware*. For in the context of dementia I think 'awareness' is more useful than the psychiatric concept of 'insight'. 'Awareness' is a concept with far greater breadth of meaning, and therefore of application. The traditional concept of 'insight' with its narrow definition is not a helpful one here, for it requires a person to admit to having made 'mistakes', and to 'feel concerned' about having made them (Jacques 1992). In other words, the person afflicted with memory loss and its concomitant confusion, who is already in a state of terrible anxiety as they realise what is happening to them, is required to make confession, to put a label on themselves, all so that they may be relegated to the ranks of those who are no longer quite 'one of us'. Far from respecting their natural desire to keep their increasing disability private, we ask them to collude in their own stigmatisation, in order (as they well know) to be banished. What we need to remember is that people with dementia have stood where 'we' now stand, but 'we' have not yet stood where they do. All the clients who spoke to me at Green House wanted very much to tell me how things were for them. They wanted to make clear to me that they *did* have awareness of themselves, their forgetfulness, their situation, their families.

'I need to be me!' is a plea for support for the person who is there *now*. We have seen that this may not be quite the same person as the one we knew 'before'. People with dementia change and evolve just like people without dementia, especially under the influence of traumatic experiences. And since we define ourselves by our cognitive abilities, what could be more traumatic than to be aware that we are losing them? So when we recognise clients' awareness we are also recognising them as individual people – and not less than any others. In acknowledging the same essence, we are supporting their personhood, their identity, their sense of self.

Sadly, many of the staff, managers and carers whom I interviewed for the original evaluation seemed unable to recognise the fact that people with dementia were not living in a state of anaesthesia. The staff justified their evaluation of clients' awareness (or not) by citing their verbal skills, and family carers did so by their ability to recognise the person they knew, and be recognised by them. Many managers admitted that they relied on staff and carers' judgements. Although there was partial recognition of clients' awareness it seemed that even those most closely involved (perhaps especially those people) were defended from a full realisation of this. The way in which their awareness was judged by others (particularly staff) in terms of their ability to make themselves understood in language had a direct effect on their experience of care. For when we believe that people are not aware, we do not interact with them in the same way. This relative lack of meaningful interaction with others has a deleterious effect on someone with dementia, who is being relegated to the world of non-persons. Is it any wonder that they become afraid, angry or withdrawn?

Awareness, of course, is a two-edged sword, for it means that a person is conscious of the bad as well as the good. Their awareness also inevitably includes awareness of losses: of faculties, home, and loved ones – through incomprehension, neglect or bereavement. How we deal with awareness of loss in people with dementia is revealing. The sort of support we would seek to provide for someone who had lost, for example, a limb, their home, or their loved ones, is denied to those with dementia. With a very few remarkable exceptions (such as Laura Sutton) we do not offer specialist counselling services to those whom neurological impairment and society have combined to deprive of their mind, their place in the world, and their family. We put them in a communal area (be it ward or 'home') with people they have never seen before, and we bathe, feed and dress them. Then, as if these were unrelated to such treatment, we note their 'symptoms' – the wandering, rocking, calling out, the aggression and the final state of apathetic withdrawal. And we switch off our usual responses to these behaviours. What would distress us if we saw it in our friends or colleagues leaves us strangely unmoved when we witness it in someone with dementia. 'It's their condition,' we say. But conditions do not get upset or angry or depressed. People do.

As individual people we each live in a subjective reality, as well as the consensus reality which we share with others. For the person with dementia the subjective world assumes greater import. This is partly as a result of the memory-impairment which eventually traps them in an eternal present, without the background information to make sense of it. But it is also the result of the refusal of those around them to enter their world other than judgementally. This was demonstrated most powerfully in the inappropriate use of 'reality orientation', where the 'reality' concerned was that of staff rather than the subjective emotional reality of clients. This was how it happened that clients' sense of loss, and especially of bereavement – their grief for lost loved ones – was answered by inappropriate reminders of the date and the passage of time, or by deflecting or diverting to other topics. To accept the reality of the client would be very painful. But unless it is accepted, clients' very real and pressing needs for emotional support and companionship along the road towards making meaning of their suffering cannot be met.

Interestingly, the Green House evaluation showed that disregard for and misunderstanding of other people's point of view was not reserved for those with dementia. It was a feature of other groups involved in the care process also. It was, indeed, an organisational phenomenon. What we might call the 'trickle-down' practice of disregard was to be seen in the sad state of relations between staff and management: 'Standards come down from the top!' Even at the outset the setting up of Green House showed that, although specifically planned and designed as part of the implementation of the community care policy, it was in fact set up against the direct and vocal opposition of the local community, who would have preferred to keep the old 'geriatric' hospital. And the evaluation interviews showed that while clients' level of awareness was largely ignored, members of the hands-on staff similarly felt unrecognised by management. In their interviews they complained not only about not being listened to, but even more vehemently about being left in ignorance of management decisions and plans which affected them: 'cloak and dagger management!' as one person graphically phrased it. Yet there was completely unnoticed irony in the parallel between their own situation and that of their clients. For when asked about clients' involvement in decisions about their own care, they saw the fact that clients' did not, in fact, participate in this as merciful, in that they thought clients would have found it too threatening. That is, they did not identify their own experience with that of their clients.

Realistically, a service which truly answers the needs of people with dementia must be based on a genuine appreciation of their awareness and experience by each and every person in the organisation involved with that service. The organisation which takes seriously the viewpoint of each of its members is a richer organisation, in that its members become full, rather than partial, members – each contributing the information which only she or he can give, and which would otherwise be lost. Each part of the organisation needs to achieve a corresponding understanding and appreciation of the viewpoint, skills, constraints and concerns of every other part. If the objective is to benefit clients, then only by garnering and harnessing its full complement of personal resources can this be achieved. Everyone – of whatever level and function – needs to be part of a continual consciousness-raising programme with regard to the subjective experience of people with dementia. The DCM project showed how important it was that such consciousness-raising should not be restricted only to hands-on staff, but should actively include strategic-level managers. For only when those who make the key decisions are both personally convinced of the awareness of people with dementia using their services, and active witnesses of the challenges facing those who deliver care, is realistic provision and support for all concerned likely to become a reality. Recognising the awareness of people with dementia has to begin with a genuine sharing of this perspective on the part of both managers and staff.

What are the resource implications here? After all, raising awareness across all personnel involved in the organisation which delivers care, and keeping that sensitivity honed, are not achieved without cost. The good news is that much of what is required is about extending existing skills, as much as learning (and evolving) new ones. It is not, for example, that we need to learn from scratch how to read people's behaviour as meaningful communication. This is something which we all already do all the time in our daily lives. Much of what we all communicate to each other in every interaction is conveyed through body language and behaviour. In actual fact the words we use are often far less important in conveying meaning to another than we think. The other person has already intuitively 'read' our body language, and if it does not agree with the substance of our words, will become uncomfortable and suspicious. This much is well known. So we have to ask why it is that when we enter a dementia care environment we switch off this natural ability: it is not that the person with dementia exists in a state of living anaesthesia, but that we consciously and deliberately anaesthetise ourselves against the meaning of what we see. To turn that switch back on is to reverse the vicious circle of denial which is our short-sighted response to the fear that encountering the other-ness of dementia arouses in us.

However, in emphasising the importance of reading non-verbal behaviour we must not discount the importance of the words that people with dementia are still able to say to us. So another resource we will need is the ability to open our ears and minds to what they are saying, receive their memory-stories, and learn to interpret their significance. Here again we will be building on existing skills, for imagination and a sensitivity for symbolism are natural human abilities, albeit too often left to atrophy. But we will need to resuscitate and cultivate them if we are to get to know the person as they are now, and to understand their subjective world so that we can enter it appropriately. To do this carries an emotional cost:

> We need to listen to the poetical, to the metaphorical aspects of the stories that people with dementia tell. But this is hard. The

stories that are told, the emotional pain that can be generated is immense. When we hear these stories we need to remember that it is not just the pain of the person with dementia that we are listening to, it is not just their losses that they are speaking of; these are also our own potential losses, our own future pain. (Sutton and Cheston 1997, p.162)

If we are to ask people to take this courageous step, therefore, we need to have something to offer in place of the short-lived, apparent emotional security which denial provided. This is why relationships of support and trust among all concerned matter so much. We need, as it were, to 'en-courage' each other by holding hands as we all turn the switch back on together. The prime resource implication, then, is a strong organisational culture of openness, trust and support, within which clinical supervision can draw out individual capabilities as it reassures individual anxieties.

But there are also considerable training implications. If we are to work facilitatively across two worlds – the subjective and the consensus reality – then this requires both sophisticated under-standing and creative interpersonal skills. This is where our inter-relating with people with dementia needs a psychotherapeutic dimension. For consensus reality can probably better be created with people with dementia by entering their world rather than insisting intransigently that they enter ours. First we need to know how to learn about the 'inner theatres' (Kets de Vries 1999) on whose stage we are the unwitting actors. This is a skilled as well as an imaginative task. And then we need to acquire the psychotherapeutic skills which will enable us to use this knowledge to advantage. This will entail the creative development of sensitive listening and counselling skills in staff members of all functions and levels. The emotional reality of individual clients must inform care practice and the quality of each interpersonal encounter, be it with domestic staff cleaning around them, the porter driving them to an appointment, the nursing assistant helping them dress, or the manager auditing the service. Most particularly there is a need for specialist counselling skills for both nursing, occupational therapy and psychology staff, especially in bereavement.

## Companionship

This brings us to the second thing the Green House experience has to contribute. For those clients with dementia who could still speak told how important to them the rest of us are. Not just as nurses, doctors or careworkers, but as people. We may not have the wonder-cure – the 'magic bullet' – which will eradicate the neurological degeneration of dementia. But right here and now we *do* possess the capability to eradicate much of the distress to which it leads. For so many of the Green House clients I interviewed, the first thing they wanted to say about the service (and the subject to which they kept returning) related to the pleasure they had in being with friendly, familiar people. And what they so valued we already have within us to give: the comfort of our companionship. But companionship is not given without cost. When we choose to 'share the darkness' (Cassidy 1988), we inevitably choose to enter it. As Henri Nouwen wrote:

> No one can help anyone without becoming involved, without entering with his whole person into the painful situation, without taking the risk of becoming hurt, wounded, or even destroyed in the process ... (without a willingness) to make one's own pain and joyful experiences available as sources of clarification and understanding ... The great illusion of leadership is to think that man can be led out of the desert by someone who has never been there. (Nouwen 1979, cited in Burnell 1989, p.72)

For clients, too, relating to others – although often so valued – carried also a cost. While they appreciated the sociability of the day-hospital, there was for them (and even more so for those in the in-patient area) a price to be paid. Part of the price was the enforced nature of their confinement with 'strange' strangers. But even for the most sociably inclined, the relationship with those who cared for them was problematic. They were grateful for the support, but the inequality of the relationship raised old, long-buried anxieties which they brought with them from the last time they were in a dependent role: in childhood. This constituted their subjective reality. Without insight into this subjective experience of dependence anyone working with people with dementia is necessarily working in the dark, like an actor pushed onto the stage, not knowing in which play they are performing. The 'doing unto' nature of so much 'care' creates this inherently undermining, unhelpful and unhealthy, one-sided relationship, which resurrects the private anguish of past helplessness. And, as the DCM observations showed, the more helpless one is, the more one is left alone in a private world of fear, resentment and despair. We need to listen to what 'care' means to any given individual with dementia, if we are going to get the relationship right. And it is relationship which the Green House clients said was so important to them.

The relationship which came most often to their mind when clients were talking about Green House was that between parent and child. And the language used and attitudes expressed by members of staff in their interviews showed that their perception of the care relationship from the opposite side, as it were, tallied completely with this metaphor of 'parentalism.' In fact, both clients and staff effectively described the care relationship, as experienced by the former and practised by the latter, as a one-way street: being taken care of, and looking after. Despite their sincere devotion to the concept of 'client-centred' care, staff left no scope for the power relationship between themselves and users of the service to be anything other than unequal. Managers also echoed this view from their own perspective. Their avowed reliance on staff for understanding clients, assessing their needs, and knowing the best way to meet those needs amounted to a picture of the omniscient parent ('mother knows best'), in the same way that clients and staff had described the omnipotent parent.

But the implication of the parental model is that it is intrinsically antagonistic to quality of care. From the clients' perspective it is inherently disempowering, contributing to self-doubt when confusion is already assailing them, and to the undermining of remaining skills – which a 'client-centred' approach is supposedly dedicated to preserving. In fact, this model also undermines in staff members individually, and the organisation in general, the motivation to be genuinely client-centred, because it is centred around the values of the deliverers of care, and not those of the recipients. This is not to say that the caregivers' values are not good ones; but they are not necessarily, and cannot be assumed to be, the same as those of the clients themselves.

In fact, all the four groups of people whom I interviewed at Green House experienced dependence on each other. We have seen how staff depended on (and felt let down by) managers, and how managers elected a dependence on staff as 'knowing best' what clients needed. One way in which the family carers demonstrated their dependence on the Green House service in particular and the health service in general was the frequent discrepancy between literal and latent meaning in their interviews. For example, while saying that they were perfectly satisfied with the service and appreciated how wonderful the staff were, they would then go on to tell stories of their experience of the service in which all had been far from wonderful: lost clothes and even lost false teeth, unexplained and disabling increases in medication, sudden worsening of nocturnal incontinence, to name but a few. That is, for the most part they only felt able to voice criticism covertly. While, of course, it is consonant with human nature for both their statements to be true without mutual invalidation, it is nevertheless also understandable that people in such great need of help (physical, emotional, psychological and financial) should be reticent about criticising the hand that feeds them. Their own suffering and desperation could not fail to colour their viewpoint.

So the perspective of each group involved with Green House was inevitably constrained by their particular state of dependence. Given this constrained perspective, how could any one group represent other than their own viewpoint? Yet both staff and managers accepted a proxy voice for the clients. Staff saw carers as the nearest approximation to the voice of the client, and managers saw staff in the same way. Yet, limited by the dependence of their own positions, neither staff nor family carers could speak for anyone other than themselves.

But no one spoke of collaborating with the clients. It was taken for granted by all the others that this was not a possibility. However, we have heard how several of the clients themselves spoke of interdependence: 'You don't have to bend down on people, not that at all, no. It's give and take. Yes, I love that – give and take.' In Chapter One I asked why we should be interested in these words of an elderly man with dementia. I think all those involved with Green House have shown us the reason. For the clients who echoed Charles were not only making a discreet plea for involvement and acceptance. They were travelling through a process of neurological deterioration which no one who has not experienced it can truly understand. They had, however, previously experienced the world without such impairment, and could therefore relate to and identify with the perspective of their relatives, the staff, and indeed myself. In other words, they were able to speak from a viewpoint which encompassed both perspectives. The rest of us, however, lacked the possibility of such a dual perspective precisely because dementia – like death – is 'the undiscover'd country, from whose bourn no traveller returns' (*Hamlet* Act 3, Scene 1, 79–80). This is why what people with dementia have to say to the rest of us is so crucially important, because it is information which we can obtain from no other source. While multidisciplinary and multiagency intercommunication and collaboration is rightly held to be a crucial feature of quality care provision, the significance of what people with dementia tell us about the value of mutual aid and interdependence lies precisely in its source: that those who have travelled to a place we cannot begin to comprehend, and of which we are all justifiably afraid, can say from those depths that what is truly important about *care* is that it should be *mutual*.

The implications of this are surely that the care process needs to include all parties. Instead of a service abrogating to itself full power over the lives of its clients, without recognising that they have a voice, and without listening to what that voice has to say, people with dementia need support provided within a framework of partnership. At Green House both staff and managers were fully cognisant of the benefits of working in partnership with family carers – although carers were not quite so aware of their value to the organisation! But the partnership needs to be extended to include the clients too. We have seen that clients both can and do work to help each other on occasion. For example, the moving instances where clients acted as advocates for one another: Norma who ensured that her friend's place was laid at table, and Jerry securing help for Joe when he was choking. And also we have seen how beneficial was the experience of working together with each other and with staff on challenging journeys in the minibus (the 'transports of delight') – although, sadly, neither the benefit nor the reason for it were noticed. We need to devise practices which proactively facilitate this sort of experience, so that clients in formal care environments have practical roles, as advocates for themselves and one another, and as true collaborators with all those with whom they are involved, either personally or organisationally. In this way, not only is the crucial input of the clients' own voice incorporated, but the personhood and well-being of each individual is supported through practical acknowledgement of their indispensability. We all need to be needed.

This was the message of the client who had been a busy wife and mother and was so anxious to find a way to help, a job to do. That there is a cost to providing care is the perennial worry of managers and policy makers. But the clients of Green House told of the cost of receiving care. To be always on the receiving end of the care relation-ship, not allowed – indeed, not considered able – to contribute, to be of value to others in their daily round, is to be shut out from the normal intercourse of human life. We need to learn the gracious art of receiving, for in caring for people with dementia it is *just* as blessed to receive as to give! Indeed, receiving is the greatest gift. People need to be needed, and to know that they are. True companionship is mutual giving and receiving.

What is needed to resource this companionship model of care? Here again we can begin by drawing on existing experience and skills. We have seen that in the DCM project, when the Green House staff in the in-patient area began to recognise the benefits which their personal interactions with their clients could bestow, they increased interaction around the activities of eating and practical physical care. But they were not able (within existing personnel and skill resources) to develop episodes of non-task-oriented interaction. This is because spending an extended period of time with someone who may not be able to communicate with us in words is perceived by most people as quite a difficult, even threatening, thing to do. We seek to structure our interactions with others around comprehensible, visible, purposeful activities, so that we (and the world of observers around us) can *know what we are doing.* This spares us from confronting the fact that we need to *just be* with others, acknowledging that it is part of being human that 'all real living is meeting' (Buber 1937).

We seem to have to justify our meetings. Yet companionship without words is something of which most of us have experience. Parents and those of a fond disposition happily spend considerable periods of time with small babies, just smiling, stroking tiny fingers, and acknowledging every coo and gurgle with admiration and delight. Lovers of all ages know the supreme satisfaction of just being able to gaze into the eyes of the beloved, holding hands and exchanging the inward, secretive smile of shared memories. Surely we have all known what it is to sit with close family or friends in front of the fire, or relaxing in the sun in the garden, when no word is, or needs to be, spoken: the companionable silence of familiarity. So we know how to do it; we just need to learn how to extend that experience into feeling comfortable and companionable with people with dementia. Of course, there are time and personnel dimensions to this too. But available person-hours can be increased, for example, by taking 'breaks' not in the staff room, but relaxing with clients. Instead of framing working with 'clients' with dementia as so stressful that we need to have time out, we might learn to think of them as people who can, and might like to be, our friends. Don't we like to have a cup of coffee with our friends?

## Counting the cost

I began this book by asking what happens to people when age and infirmity, rather than affection and shared interest, shape relationships between them. Listening to *all* those involved at Green House tells us about the costs of care in the present inadequate system.

Demographic changes and the twilight of the welfare state have led to the question of how to fund long-term care for the elderly as a high priority on the social policy agenda. There is much concern about the costs of care. But who would look at cost without looking at what they are buying? The 'what' and 'how' of care cannot be separated from discussions of cost. At present, across both public and private sectors, we devote enormous financial resources to a system of care for older people with dementia which perhaps keeps some people warm, clothed and fed, but also delivers massive stresses and strains to over-stretched care staff, relatives too desperate to complain, and caught-in-the-middle managers. And the elderly clients with dementia may be warm and clothed and fed, but they are also left alone in their distress – and the greater this becomes, the more they are left alone. Is this really 'value for money'?

Cost needs to be understood as not just financial, but also psychological and emotional. The difficulty is that money can be counted, while feelings cannot. But just because you can count something does not mean that you have found what you need to be concentrating on. 'Countability' is not the defining feature of a cost. Einstein said that 'not everything that can be counted counts, and not everything that counts can be counted.' Abraham Kaplan went even further when he wrote that 'if you can measure it, that ain't it!' (in Berg 1989, p.2). While responsible stewardship of limited public resources is greatly to be desired, the crusade for cost-effectiveness can degenerate into an inappropriately blinkered concentration on the letter of the law, when all that is taken into consideration is the financial cost of providing a service. We may try to quantify stress in terms of sick-leave and staff turnover, but that does not begin to show us the dimensions of the suffering experienced. And while, in its own way, DCM has given us a rough guide to quantifying the well- and ill-being of people with dementia, even that cannot begin to convey the depth of desperation in them that any of us can encounter if we trouble to stop, look and listen. 'My problem is myself. I got to go round here on my own, don't matter who is with me,' said James. The greatest costs are borne in largest measure by the most vulnerable: the very people for whom the services are ostensibly provided.

It is precisely by *not* listening, by denying the subjective reality of someone with dementia and insisting on our own consensus reality, that we become part of the process by which that subjective reality completely takes over. That is, by not sharing it, by not extending our ears and our imagination, we become part of the 'de-menting' process. The memory-stories are always being told, the behaviour is always there to be read (the wandering, rocking, calling out). Missed opportunities are the 'opportunity costs' of not getting things right. For Green House shows us that it is not impossible to access the perspective, the views and the experience of people with dementia, so that they may be included in the decisions which affect them. It has shown that even severely handicapped clients are still aware of themselves and their situation, and, what is more, that they are able to communicate their viewpoint and concerns. It has also shown how fundamental these concerns are, and how profound the insights which they have to offer. That is, not only do clients have a voice, but what they have to say is important. To ignore these voices is to forego a crucial input for both service design and care practice. It is also to discount the testimony that they give about the costs of receiving care when services are designed uniquely from the providers' perspective. For when care is a one-way street it is an exercise of power, no matter how well-intentioned. In proceeding solely from the perspective of all those involved in the service who do *not* have dementia, a terrible cost is paid in unanswered fear and frustration, and unconsoled depression and grief – and it is paid by thousands of elderly people already prey to physical frailty and incapacitating cognitive disruption.

Correspondingly, it needs to be recognised that there are also significant costs to working in the dark. To spend each working day face-to-face with the emotional pain and the desperation of elderly clients with a 'de-menting illness' whose causation and process remain largely mysterious, and for which no real medico-chemical solutions are at hand, can be a draining experience of disempowerment and despair. To manage such services, or their support, often with little understanding of the nature and therefore the needs of the clients, but eternally squeezed between diminishing financial resources on the one hand and the clamour of over-stressed staff on the other, can likewise be a recipe for cynicism and despair. So a heavy psychological and emotional price is also paid by staff and managers. Family carers, too, are separated from their client relative by a gulf of misperception, often alienated from the life of the community around them, and too desperately grateful for whatever service is provided to feel able and free to honestly voice their concerns. And what, we might ask, have been the opportunity costs of working in the dark? What has not been achieved owing to the absence of the perspective of the clients themselves? What might we have achieved by now if we had used this crucial input? How much effort, enthusiasm and energy has been expended on providing services which do not address the actual, profound needs of people with dementia, as they themselves see them? The story of Green House was one of much effort, enthusiasm and energy – but where it did benefit clients the most, this was not recognised, and it left its most disabled clients with the least support.

Was it a ledger around which Frans Hals' regents and regentesses grouped themselves? I strongly suspect that it was, for that was what they were concerned with: the proper administration of alms to the frail and destitute elderly. They were, of course, not wrong to place a high value on the stewardship of public funds. But in the twenty-first century it is time that we think also of another sort of stewardship, of moral obligation, towards the community and its resources. That is the duty we owe to one another to support the emotional and psychological well-being of all of us involved in the process of caring for people who need our help. This book has emphasised the priority we should accord to the perspective of elderly clients with dementia. This was in large measure because the balance of historical neglect needs to be redressed. But the Green House evaluation shows us that the well-being of clients is intimately connected with the well-being of staff, family carers and managers.

When Norma said 'I need to be me!' she was expressing the most profound emotional and psychological need that any of us (in our culture) has: to be able to retain a sense of our individual, unique and irreplaceable self. And that need is especially keen for those whose degenerative brain disorder is robbing them of a secure memory-trail for their identity. Those who accompany them need to continually reprovide the wherewithal for a secure sense of self in each present moment. This is a demanding requirement. And so, in our concern to support the personhood and well-being of each individual elderly person with dementia in our care services, we need to remember that this will necessarily entail supporting the personhood and well-being of all those who are involved with them. The care process is a web of personal and organisational interconnections. As Samuel said: 'We all rely on one another.'

# References

Barnett, E. (1997) 'Collaboration and interdependence: care as a two-way street.' In M. Marshall (ed) *State of the Art in Dementia Care*. London: Centre for Policy on Ageing.

Barthes, R. (1964) *Elements of Semiology*. New York: Hill and Wang

Berg, B.L. (1989) *Qualitative Research Methods for the Social Sciences*. Boston: Allyn & Bacon.

Buber, M. (1937) *I and Thou*, trans. R. Gregor Smith. Edinburgh: Clark.

Burnell, S.J. (1989) *Broken for Life*. London: Quaker Home Service.

Cassidy, S. (1988) *Sharing the Darkness*. London: Darton, Longman & Todd.

Collis, J.S. (1972) *The Vision of Glory*. London: C. Knight.

Conway, M.A. (1990) *Autobiographical Memory: an Introduction*. Milton Keynes: Open University Press.

Douglas, J.D. (1985) *Creative Interviewing*. London: Sage Library for Social Research.

Gibson, F. (1999) 'Can we risk person-centred communication?' *Journal of Dementia Care 7*, 5, 20–24.

Goldsmith, M. (1996) *Hearing the Voice of People with Dementia*. London: Jessica Kingsley Publishers.

Hogg, M.A. and Vaughan, G.M. (1995) *Social Psychology: an Introduction*. Hemel Hempstead: Prentice Hall/Harvester Wheatsheaf.

Holden, U. and Woods, R.T. (1995) *Positive Approaches to Dementia Care* (3rd ed). New York: Churchill Livingstone.

Hwang, D.H. (1989) *1000 Airplanes on the Roof*. Layton, UT: Gibbs Smith.

Jacques, A. (1992) *Understanding Dementia* (2nd ed). Edinburgh: Churchill Livingstone.

Jones, G. and Miesen, B.M.L. (eds.) (1992) *Care-Giving in Dementia: Research and Applications*. London: Routledge.

Kets de Vries, M.F.R. (1999) 'What's playing in the organisational theatre? Collusive relationships in management.' *Human Relations 52*, 6, 745–773.

Kitwood, T. (1990) 'The dialectics of dementia.' *Ageing and Society 10*, 177–196.

Kitwood, T. (1995) 'Positive long-term changes in dementia.' *Journal of Mental Health 4*, 133–144.

Kitwood, T. (1997) *Dementia Reconsidered: the Person Comes First*. Buckingham: Open University Press.

Kitwood, T. and Benson, S. (eds.) (1995) *The New Culture of Dementia Care*. London: Hawker Publications.

Kitwood, T. and Bredin, K. (1994) *Evaluating Dementia Care: the Dementia Care Mapping Method.* Bradford: Bradford University Dementia Group.

Le Guin, U. (1989) *Dancing at the Edge of the World.* London: Victor Gollancz.

Marshall, M. (ed.) (1997) *State of the Art in Dementia Care.* London: Centre for Policy on Ageing.

Miesen, B. (1992) 'Attachment theory and dementia.' In G. Jones and B. M. L. Miesen (eds) *Care-Giving in Dementia:* Research and Applications. London: Routledge.

Mishler, E.G. (1986) *Research Interviewing.* Cambridge, MA: Harvard University Press.

Netten, A. (1993) *A Positive Environment?* Aldershot: Ashgate.

Nouwen, H.J.M. (1979) *The Wounded Healer.* New York: Doublay.

Polanyi, M. (1966) *The Tacit Dimension.* London: Routledge A. Kegan Paul.

Ricoeur, P. (1976) *Interpretation Theory: Discourse and the Surplus of Meaning.* Houston, TX: Texas Christian University Press.

Sacks, O. (1985) *The Man Who Mistook His Wife For A Hat.* London: Picador.

de Saussure, F. (1974) *Course in General Linguistics.* London: Fontana.

Seebohm, F. (Chairman) (1968) *Report of the Committee on Local Authority and allied Social Services.* Cmnd 3703. London: HMSO

Segal, S.P. and Baumohl, J. (1988) 'No place like home: reflections on sheltering a diverse population.' In C.J. Smith and J.A. Giggs (eds) *Location and Stigma: Contemporary Perspectives on Mental Health and Mental Health Care.* London: Unwin Hyman.

Shotter, J. (1993) *Conversational Realities: Constructing Life through Language.* London: Sage.

Sixsmith, A., Stilwell, J. and Copeland, J. (1993) 'Rementia: challenging the limits of dementia care.' *International Journal of Geriatric Psychiatry 8,* 993–1000.

Sutton, L. (1993) 'The psychology of memory and meaning; a revision for a reorientation to elderly mental health.' Unpublished article; personal communication with the author.

Sutton, L. and Fincham, F. (1994) 'Clients' perspectives: experiences of respite care.' *PSIGE Newsletter 49,* 12–15.

Sutton, L. and Hopkins, V. (1994) 'Dementia in acute units; communication.' *Nursing Standard 9,* 4, 25–26.

Sutton, L.J. and Cheston, R. (1997) 'Rewriting the story of dementia: a narrative approach to psychotherapy with people with dementia.' In M. Marshall (ed) *State of the Art in Dementia Care.* London: Centre for Policy on Ageing

Titmus, R.M. (1961) 'Community care: Fact or Fiction?' Reprinted in *Commitment to Welfare.* London: Allen and Unwin 1968.

Townsend, P. (1962) *The Last Refuge: A Summary of Residential institutions and Homes for the Aged in England and Wales.* London: Routledge and Kegan Paul.

# Subject Index

abilities
  loss of, and quality of care 153
  range of in 'dementia' 49–50
  verbal, and levels of well-being and ill-being 15, 50, 131–40, 147, 150, 153
accountability 12
Adult Community Mental Health Team 69
advocacy, limits of 179
age
  reason for forgetfulness 122
  and recognition 89–91
agency, sense of 58
Alzheimer's disease 30, 31
anger, parental memories of 118
'asylums' 30
  reprovision programme 67, 68
attachment theory 117
autobiographical life-review 90, 91–94
awareness, people with dementia's 12, 14, 31–32, 128–29
  of approaching death 88–89, 161–62
  carers' view of 162–64
  changing 95–97
  communicative ability 109, 131–40, 153, 159–60, 178, 202
  denying 33–34
  and experience of care 131–40
  identity and recognition 91–95, 125
  imaginative identification 178
  of interview 82–85
  level of dependence 150–51, 153

managers' view of 158–60
meaning of concept 201
of own confusion 86–88
and punishment 136
recognition of 162, 177, 178, 184–90, 201–7, 202
staff's view of 158–60

behaviour
  disapproval of 22
  as meaningful communication 14, 16, 39, 64, 130, 189, 205
  'problems' 35
Behaviour Category Codes 58, 59
  comparison between evaluation and DCM project 188, 191–92
  highest scoring 133
bereavement 112–14, 118, 148–49, 169, 170, 194, 203
body language, listening to 64, 189, 205
buildings, inappropriate design for clients 116, 158–59, 163, 166, 174

Capital and Estates Department 69–70, 72, 75
capital programmes 79
'care in the community' see community care
care relationship, depicted by Frans Hals 18 illus., 19–20, 154, 200
care styles, and clients' ability to communicate 138–40, 139gr.
Care Values 56, 58, 59, 61
  comparison between evaluation and DCM project 186–87, 187gr., 196
  improvement in average, in DCM project 185–86, 185gr.
  mathematical problems of 61
carers
  dependence 175–77, 209–10

relationship with staff 160
viewed as voice of people with dementia 160, 166, 175
views of 157–58, 162–64, 167–68, 170–71, 174–77
change, process of 189, 196
'charity' 20
childhood memories 26
'client-centred' care 67, 160, 208–9
clients *versus* patients 153
cognitive abilities, as defining characteristic of humans 33–34
communication 13, 24–25, 37
  accessing emotional functioning 42
  between carers and service 176
  commonality of experience 100–101
  erecting barriers 21
  establishing 23
  familiarity 101–3, 165–66
  friendship 100
  interviewing technique 39, 40
  levels of 53
  loneliness 108–9
  medical model of dementia 129
  in planning and implementation 66
  preserving identity 102
  risking person-centred 20–21
  staff and management 78
  training of staff 34–35
  understanding the process 43–45
  using imagination and intuition 50
  verbal ability, and levels of well-being and ill-being 15, 50, 131–40, 147, 150, 153
community, disregarding wishes of 79–80
community care 31, 68, 103
  Health Service reforms 79
  problems of 67

# Author Index